EXTRAORDINARY CHINESE MEDICINE

EXTRAORDINARY CHINESE MEDICINE

The Extraordinary Vessels, Extraordinary Organs, and the Art of Being Human

THOMAS RICHARDSON

with William Morris

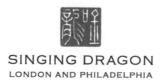

SINGING DRAGON

LONDON AND PHILADELPHIA

Quotations from *The Eight Extraordinary Meridians*, Claude Larre and Elisabeth Rochet de la Vallée [transcribed and edited by Sandra Hill], Monkey Press, London, 1997, are reproduced with kind permission from Monkey Press.

The Appendix charts are reproduced from *Chinese Medical Qigong Therapy* (2000) by Jerry Alan Johnson by kind permission of Dr. Jerry Alan Johnson.

First published in 2018
by Singing Dragon
an imprint of Jessica Kingsley Publishers
73 Collier Street
London N1 9BE, UK
and
400 Market Street, Suite 400
Philadelphia, PA 19106, USA

www.singingdragon.com

Copyright © Thomas Richardson 2018
Foreword copyright © William Morris 2018

Library of Congress Cataloging in Publication Data
A CIP catalog record for this book is available from the Library of Congress

British Library Cataloguing in Publication Data
A CIP catalogue record for this book is available from the British Library

ISBN 978 1 84819 419 9
eISBN 978 0 85701 371 2

Printed and bound by CPI Group (UK) Ltd, Croydon, CR0 4YY

CONTENTS

Foreword

For starters, I believe this book presents groundbreaking material, rooted in good Chinese medical thought. Not reproductive knowledge, but rather this is a creative piece which possesses the spark of genius. I am not certain which day the muse visited Thomas, but it clearly took place.

I see this book as part of the second wave of conscious evolutionary work in Chinese medicine in the West. The first was when this medicine exploded in the USA during the 1970s. Then the field dug into translational work, building knowledge, credibility, and improvement of the educational systems for Chinese medicine in the United States. These developments have led us to this juncture where syncretic works like this are a possibility.

Thomas and I met in the spring of 2006. The setting: a school of Chinese medicine surrounded by koi, lilies, a gazebo, a bridge, and oak trees. It was an environment conducive to inspired dialog, and our musings wandered over the matters of theory and practice.

While I served as president, I was insistent that I keep my skills as a practitioner and teacher. Thus, Thomas and I worked together in the clinic and the classroom. He attended my intensives on pulse diagnosis and eventually assisted. Upon leaving school, his practice was immediately successful.

I developed insight into mentor–mentee relations while attending the University of Southern California program on medical education. The program director's research area was mentor–mentee relations. The core factor in the process is that the mentor has to ensure the safe harbor of the relationship as the mentee attains professional standing and makes contributions to the field. This experience sensitized me to the need to nurture and support my relationship with Thomas, which has proven fruitful, as can be seen by the contents of this book.

Before turning to this book and Thomas's work, in particular, I would like to situate the conversation into an American history of acupuncture since this syncretic work is that of a white male practicing in the USA.

Benjamin Franklin's great-grandson was one Dr. Franklin Bache, who was born in Monticello, Virginia, in 1801. He graduated from the medical department at the University of Pennsylvania in 1823, ultimately serving as medical director and Commodore for the US Navy. Franklin Bache had a great passion for acupuncture, gaining access to the French practitioners who brought the practices back to Europe. He actively promoted acupuncture and its research early in his career circa 1825.

By the end of the 19th century, one of the four founding professors of Johns Hopkins Hospital, a Canadian by the name of Sir William Osler, promoted the use of acupuncture for lumbago. He further developed an appreciation for acupuncture and Chinese medical thought among the Johns Hopkins community in his lecture series which became the book *Practice of Medicine*, published in 1897.

As the story goes, in 1971, James Reston, a reporter for *The New York Times*, received surgery for appendicitis while on Nixon's China trip. His postoperative pain was relieved by acupuncture at the Anti-Imperialist Hospital in Beijing. Nixon's physician, Dr. Walter Tkach, was so impressed with the treatments he saw in China that he encouraged the National Institutes of Health to set up the Ad Hoc Committee on Acupuncture, with an acupuncture research conference held the following year. The high-level governmental focus on acupuncture created a wave of interest, whereby research began at Los Angeles medical schools at the University of Southern California and University of California, Los Angeles (UCLA). That interest soon faded as the physician-researchers untrained in acupuncture had difficulty getting it to work. These activities were a prelude to the advent of schools for acupuncture shortly to come.

Dr. Homer Chang chartered the Sino-American Rehabilitation Association in 1969 which became SAMRA University and operated as a training center for Traditional Chinese Medicine (TCM) missionaries in 1972. A little later, a group of disbanded researchers from UCLA gathered under James Tin Yau So in Boston to form the first state-approved acupuncture school at the New England School of Acupuncture in 1974.

During the "decade of unrest," acupuncture exploded into the consciousness of northern Americans. Youth experimented with mind expansion through chemicals and meditative practices. The idea of acupuncture enfolded into a period focused on conscious evolution.

The wave of acupuncture as a discipline in the West gained licensure, and in 1996 the US Food and Drug Administration reclassified acupuncture needles from the investigative category to an "accepted medical instrument." These changes led to another explosion of acupuncture and, subsequently, more focus upon translation of texts and a further professionalization of the practice.

Arriving now at the current moment, I believe the practice of acupuncture as an American discipline is experiencing a recursion of the spiritual impact of acupuncture, and Thomas Richardson is an agent of this social movement as medicine.

When Thomas introduced his idea about connecting the eight extraordinary vessels with the cycling of nutrient *qi*, his palpable excitement struck me fast and hard. I made a determined effort to encourage the inspiration Thomas expressed. I encouraged him to root the citations within the Han Dynasty lore, which provide the canonical locus of such thought. He pursued that recommended focus, and throughout the years I have participated with him in his creative explorations of this work.

Thomas engages creative inquiry with passion and discipline. I wanted to encourage his creative efforts, as Chinese medicine in the West often takes on the values of direct translation and accurate reproduction of the knowledge transmissions across cultures. Contrarily, creative inquiry requires discipline, which requires operating from a transdisciplinary perspective.

Extraordinary Chinese Medicine is a pearl ground in the currents of inspiration, literate discourse, and practice. The poetic passages drew me in, and the images explicate deep problems of theory with beauty.

This book presents a refreshing exercise born of realization. It is a powerful book borne of the internal practices that Thomas has engaged in combination with his continued studies of Daoist thought at Harvard University. This bricolage has brought new perspectives upon the problems of theory and practice in Chinese medicine. The ideas contained herein are rooted in classical lore and as such bear the imprint of a research discipline that I call "contemplative hermeneutics." Distinct from a hermeneutics of contemplation, where the study focuses upon materials arising during a meditative state, *contemplative hermeneutics* denotes the focus upon textual passages during contemplation.

The *contemplative hermeneutical* practices in which Thomas has engaged to develop the contents of this book take place at the intersection of contemporary practice, Daoist thought, and the Han Dynasty canonical lore, thus qualifying this book as a *transdisciplinary* effort.

Thus, Thomas has approached this book with rigor, openness, and tolerance. He has expressed rigor in his thesis, taking into account existing information in the field and exploring the resources available at Harvard, and his openness demonstrates an acceptance of the unknown, the unexpected, and the unforeseeable.

William Morris, PhD, DAOM
February 2018, British Colombia

Acknowledgments

This book began as a series of articles, and I am extraordinarily grateful to many individuals who read, edited, and made comments and suggestions during these early stages. In particular, I am grateful to Steve Clavey and *The Lantern*, and Attilio D'Alberto and *Chinese Medicine Times*, for publishing many of these articles, as well as offering edits, comments and suggestions, and other directions and books to investigate.[1] Likewise, I am grateful to the editors and staff at *The American Acupuncturist*, *Acupuncture Today*, *The Empty Vessel*, and *California Journal of Oriental Medicine*, for publishing articles and content related to this work, and to Doan Ky for reading and editing many of the early articles.[2]

I owe a debt of gratitude to Michael Corner for his graphic design work, and for turning my rough drawings into the figures that you see in this book. To Jessica Kingsley and the staff at Singing Dragon, I am extremely thankful for all of their help in bringing this project to fruition.

1 See Richardson 2010a, 2010b, 2010c, 2011, 2012a, 2012b, and 2014.
2 See Richardson 2008, 2009a, 2009b, and 2015.

I am also grateful to Janet Gyatso, my advisor at Harvard Divinity School, who oversaw the independent study which eventually became Chapter 1 on the natural state— her guidance and editing were indispensable in the research and writing of this material.

I am grateful to my parents for their continued encouragement and support, and to Heather Brassell, for encouraging me to pick this work up again and finish it after it lay dormant for several years. I am also very grateful to the many teachers, practitioners, and scholars in the history of Chinese medicine upon whose shoulders this work stands, and to the body of work they have created over the last several thousand years to which I hope this may make some small, modest contribution. And lastly, I am grateful to William Morris for being an amazing mentor and tireless support, teacher, and friend throughout the years, for spending so much time editing, reviewing, and commenting on these ideas and this work as it has unfolded over the last decade, and for continually inspiring me to learn and grow as a practitioner, scholar, and writer.

PREFACE

When I began studying acupuncture and Oriental medicine at the Academy of Oriental Medicine at Austin (AOMA) Graduate School of Integrative Medicine, I quickly fell in love with it. For the first time in my life, I felt as if I had been given a user's manual for this body that I had been using (and abusing) for 25 years. It was a user's manual not only for the body, but for the emotions, the mind, and the spirit. It was amazing to see how connected everything is, and how by simply pushing (or needling) a point on my body I could instantaneously change what I was feeling physically and emotionally, that I was able to instantly shift my state of consciousness. At the same time that I began studying Oriental medicine, I began practicing *qigong* and meditation intensively for the first time in my life. For several years, I was practicing *qigong*, yoga, and meditation for 4–5 hours a day, at the same time as I was learning the acupuncture points and channels.

This naturally developed into using the points and channels as a focus of meditation and *qigong*—not only as a means of shifting my state of consciousness but also (and perhaps more practically) as a means of studying. I began to study and memorize the points by bringing my awareness into and through the points one at a time, while repeating (verbally or silently in my mind) the point categories and primary functions and uses of each point. Most often I would follow the daily flow of *ying qi* in the primary channels— starting in the Lung channel with *zhongfu* LU-1, moving to *yunmen* LU-2, and all the way down to *shaoshang* LU-11, and then moving into the Large Intestine channel and traveling from *shangyang* LI-1 all the way up to *yingxiang* LI-20, and from there into the Stomach channel, and so forth. More nights than I can count, I fell asleep to this meditation of feeling the flow of *qi* through the primary channels while reviewing the points. As time went on, this helped me to heal and balance myself on many different levels, and it also led to many insights into the placement of the various acupuncture points, their associated categories, and their functions.

One day during this period of time, I went out for a run. As I was running, I decided to begin this meditation on the flow of *qi* through the channels. Soon after starting at the beginning of the Lung channel, I reached *lieque* LU-7. As my awareness moved into the point, I thought to myself, "*Luo*-connecting point. Command point for the back of the head and nape of the neck. Confluent point of the *ren mai*." As soon as I thought, "Confluent point of the *ren mai*," I felt the entire pathway of the *ren mai* light up within my body (see the Appendix for a chart showing the pathway of the *ren mai*). I suddenly became curious about what order the other extraordinary vessels would be activated as I followed the flow of *qi* through the primary channels, and from there this work was born. I realized that there was a deep connection between the flow of *qi* through the primary channels, the placement of the confluent points of the extraordinary vessels along the primary channel system, and Daoist conceptions of the evolution of consciousness.

Being a student at the time, and not having very much depth or experience with the classics of Chinese medicine, I was not sure if what I had stumbled upon had already been written, or if it was actually meaningful, or if it was really nothing at all. The next day in clinic, I shared some of what I had experienced with Will Morris, my clinic supervisor and mentor. He immediately replied enthusiastically that I should put it down on paper, and write an article about it. And so I did, and he graciously edited it, as well as suggesting which parts needed more support (and where to look for such support), and what parts may be a bit of a stretch. That was the beginning.

The more I began researching these relationships, the more other aspects revealed themselves to me—including direct relationships between the extraordinary vessels and the extraordinary *fu*, as well as direct relationships to the primary channels and *zangfu* organs themselves. But more than anything, what became clear is that the entire channel system demonstrates a deep, underlying, and continuous connection between the individual and their environment, a continuous connection to Heaven above and Earth below, and, perhaps most importantly, an underlying drive of the channel systems to continually, experientially bring us back to the transcendent unity that we are always a part of. While I had understood for a long time that the body has an innate capacity to heal, what became clear is that there is also an innate drive to return to the natural state and to experience unity, even while existing as individuated humans at the level of duality.

As all of this work unfolded, eventually becoming a series of many articles over multiple years, Will was always there—guiding, editing, suggesting, and giving constructive criticism. He offered a perfect balance of support while lending a critical eye of wisdom and insight gained from decades of working with this medicine. Without Will's help, support, and guidance, none of this would have been possible, and I am eternally grateful to him for graciously spending so much of his precious time to work with me on this project that I am so passionate about and inspired by. He has been the greatest mentor I could have asked for, and this work is what it is because of him.

INTRODUCTION

Life is extraordinary. Life is never static; it constantly moves, transforms, and evolves. At times smoothly, seamlessly, while at other times drastically, even seemingly catastrophically. Throughout it all, however, there is always an inherent integrity present, underlying it all, holding it all together, and assisting in the times of transformation and evolution. Within the human body, the eight extraordinary vessels (*qi jing ba mai* 奇經八脈) are a direct reflection of this simultaneous oneness, multidimensionality, integration, and transformation that is an integral part of life.

At the level of humanity, we exist in duality, yet we are inherently connected to, and constantly strive to experience, unity. The practice of medicine is the art of healing, the art of "making whole"—this refers to becoming whole not only at the micro level (within self) but also at a macro level (the connection between the individual and the rest of existence). This is also the art of humanity, to experience wholeness within self and connection to Heaven above, Earth below, and to all that exists at the level of manifest reality. When the *qi* flows freely through the body, *yin* and *yang*, Heaven and Earth, inside and outside, and body and spirit are smoothly integrated into one dynamic, unified state of being; thus duality is transcended and the state of oneness can be experienced within self. This is a state of being, a state of experiential awareness, which can be contrasted with various states where the *qi* does not flow freely through the body (e.g. when blockages exist), and one experiences a sense of separation.

The experience and act of transcending duality, of experiencing unity, is truly extraordinary. In fact, it is precisely the moments of transcendence within life that make life extraordinary, that bring meaning to life. Whether we call the all-pervading presence the *dao*, God, Absolute Oneness, or any other term, what we are often referring to is the underlying unity that creates a continuity from one moment in time to the next, from one physical space to another. This presence transcends the dualities of time and space, and creates continuity across all dimensions of being and experience; by the very nature that it transcends duality, it cannot be grasped or truly understood through the mind. It is this all-pervading presence which experientially allows each individuated being to connect to all else that is present, and thus to live and exist in the natural state.

Throughout history, many cultures have seen an overlap between spiritual practices, healing practices, and medical practice, and the physician was often considered a holy person within the community and vice versa. There may be numerous reasons for this, but I believe one of the primary reasons to be that the intent and aim of both spiritual practices and the practice of medicine is to assist in making us whole, to help us transcend the limitedness of duality and rediscover this natural state of wholeness and connectedness.

When a patient comes in with a primary complaint or imbalance, simply treating the symptoms is often enough to make them feel more comfortable. However, when the underlying imbalance that gave rise to the manifest symptoms begins to resolve, it is the patient themselves, and not simply the symptom, that begins to shift. It is a change of their perspective, how they view themselves and the world around them, and it changes their experience of reality. In other words, it is a shift of consciousness. And whenever consciousness shifts towards a greater state of unity, it is an experience that transcends the mundane. Similarly, many spiritual practices have such a shift of consciousness as either a goal or a direct effect. Whether it is prayer, yoga, meditation, *qigong*, chanting, or ritual, all of these tend to lead to a shift in the consciousness of the individuals involved, and often it is a shift that helps them feel more integrated within self as well as more connected to something transcendent, to something that transcends the limited, individuated self. It is this shift in awareness that leads one to feel re-connected to something divine, to the all-pervading presence.

When there are blockages within the body—whether energetic, physical, emotional, mental, or otherwise—then one feels disconnected, dis-integrated, and therefore one does not feel whole. It is when these blockages are removed and the *qi* flows freely through the body that integration, healing, and connection can occur, for it is only through the *qi* flowing freely that body and spirit can be completely integrated with each other. Thus, with the removal of each blockage, the individual moves closer to being whole, and heals at a new level. Such moments of healing are extraordinary experiences, because they bring us successively closer to the natural state, where we are more completely connected within self as well as connected to Heaven above, Earth below, and the world around us.

＊ ＊ ＊

In this book, I examine relationships between Daoism and Chinese medicine, and in particular the ways in which the extraordinary vessels may be considered "extraordinary" precisely because they enable us to call up the reserves necessary to reconnect to the knowledge and experience of oneness within ourselves. I also propose a model that expands upon the existing body of theoretical knowledge in Chinese medicine by examining ways in which the extraordinary vessels and the extraordinary organs may be deeply and intimately connected to each other as well as the primary channels and *zangfu*. Through such connections, they create opportunities for us to transcend duality and the mundane reality and reconnect with the ever-present, all-pervading unity, allowing one to be more fully, experientially present.

Within the meridian system, the primary meridians correspond relatively more to duality and the mundane reality; thus they are organized into *yin–yang* pairs and relate to the daily functioning of the body. On the other hand, the extraordinary vessels exemplify the process and experience of transcendence, the shift of consciousness that occurs in both healing and spiritual practice, and correspond more to oneness. For this reason, the extraordinary vessels have often been used for various Daoist spiritual practices, meditations, and *qigong*, and this is due, in part, to the ability of the extraordinary vessels to effect deeper, transcendent healing within self and with patients.

What I offer in this book is a theoretical model that examines the ways in which the extraordinary vessels and the extraordinary organs have relationships to Daoist cosmology, and the ways in which they may have relationships to the transcendent, creative, spiritual, mystical, and extraordinary aspects of humanity. This model is simply another way of organizing information on the extraordinary vessels and organs—and their relationships to the primary channels and *zangfu*—in a manner that creates a new perspective; it is my hope that this perspective may enable a fuller understanding of the ways in which these vessels function. As with all perspectives and models, it has its limitations, and is not meant to be something that is applied all the time, in all cases. However, I do believe that it has a great deal of usefulness, not only in presenting a framework for gaining a theoretical understanding of the extraordinary vessels and the extraordinary organs and their relation to the primary channel and *zangfu* organ systems, but more importantly for affecting the way in which we perceive the individual patient that presents to us in clinic. My hope and intent is that this model will inform the perspective and internal state of practitioners—the way in which they see themselves, their patients, and this beautiful, extraordinary medicine that we work with.

It is important to state at the outset that this is not a clinical manual, per se. Within these pages you will not find defined treatment protocols or guidelines of what points to use, in which order, for various imbalances. Nor will you find detailed presentations of each of the extraordinary vessels.

While there is some discussion of acupuncture points and their uses, this is intended primarily to illustrate some of the theories and principles found within these pages. The reasons for this are simple. First, information and presentations of the extraordinary vessel pathways and points can be found elsewhere in various books from the classics to more contemporary authors. Second, it is my belief that medicine in general, and acupuncture in particular, is more of an art than a science—even while having characteristics of both. But when it comes to the individual practitioner practicing the medicine, they are practicing an art. And any art form, by nature, is an expression of the artist's perspective and sense of humanity and the cosmos. Art is an external expression of what is experienced internally; it is creativity that transcends the mundane and leads to the extraordinary moments of life. As written in the Bhagavad Gita, "It is better to walk one's own path poorly, than to walk another's path exquisitely." I have no desire to give treatment protocols for others to practice by rote; I prefer to share a perspective that may be of use as each practitioner practices this art of medicine in their own independent, fully embodied way.

Therefore, what you will find in the following chapters is a perspective, a way of organizing information, a way of seeing—of seeing yourself, your patients, the medicine, and the interaction between these various aspects. It is a perspective that sees each individual as inextricably linked to Heaven and Earth, as well as to their environment and others around them. A perspective that sees medicine as a practice that not only helps to alleviate suffering, but also has the capacity to enable each individual to live a more fully developed and actualized life, to move through life's trials with a greater degree of grace, understanding, growth, and wisdom, and that can be utilized to help patients move closer to the natural state, towards a greater degree of enlightenment. One of the extraordinary aspects of Chinese medicine is that it is a medical model that still offers a relatively integrated perspective of the various aspects of humanity—including physical, emotional, mental, social, and spiritual—and is thus aptly suited for treating everything from physical injuries to spiritual crises, as well as for seeing the connection between seemingly disparate afflictions and imbalances.

A fundamental component of this viewpoint is the assumption that the art of medicine cannot be separated from some form of transcendent perspective—whether it be simply a sense of interconnectedness or a more fully developed cosmology/spirituality/religion—without often becoming dehumanizing, or at the very least not being as capable of helping individuals to live more actualized lives. This is not intended as a condemnation of practitioners or patients who do not have a spiritual belief structure or spiritual practice, nor is it intended as a directive that one must be spiritual to practice medicine. It is simply an acknowledgment that any institution that deals with the fundamental questions of humanity—whether it be medicine, economics, education, or other—will have a tendency to become dehumanizing if it is not informed by a model or perspective that can account for all of the various dynamic aspects of humanity—particularly the physical, emotional, mental, social, and spiritual.

Herbs, acupuncture, bodywork, dietary therapy, and *qigong*, as well as pharmaceutical agents and surgery, are all methods that can be employed to help "fix" imbalances in the individual. What may be even more important, *a priori*, is the internal state of the individual who applies any of these methods—the practitioner's own humanity, and cultivating this humanity so that we can be more fully present—and compassionate—with our patients. In being more fully present with them, we can help patients to be more present with themselves, which will increase the effectiveness of all of the other treatment modalities that we employ. For example, acupuncture can be very effective for a large number of complaints; however, when the patient is able to relax and be more fully present with the needles in, and bring more awareness into their body, the effectiveness and outcomes of treatment improve dramatically. Presence is like a magnet; the more present one is, the more it enables others to become more present.

I also tend to find that there are few things in this world that do as much damage to the human condition as guilt. It is for this reason that I try to refrain from being dogmatic with patients, and similarly I will attempt to refrain from being dogmatic in presenting this theoretical perspective. This is merely one perspective, one lens through which to view the All, and it is certainly not absolute. As the first line of the *Dao De Jing* states, "The *dao* that can be spoken is not the eternal and everlasting *dao*." I therefore encourage other practitioners and students to use the information and perspective found herein when it is appropriate and helpful, and cast it aside when it is not. This is one of the beautiful aspects of Oriental medicine, and of medicine as a whole—there are unlimited overlapping and often contradictory perspectives and ways of viewing humanity, and we can shift lenses whenever it seems appropriate based upon the presenting patient and their condition, as well as our own personal state of consciousness at any given moment. This is an integral part of practicing the art of medicine. Each perspective and theory is a tool, a color of paint, to be brought in or switched out when necessary, but never to become the sole tool or color that one uses. After all, as the saying goes, if all you have is a hammer, everything starts to look like a nail.

*   *   *

As stated above, I view the practice of medicine as both an art and a science.[1] We study and learn the system so that when the time comes to apply it there is a greater possibility of successfully helping others. Yet no matter how much one studies, no matter how well one knows the science of any given medical system, there always remain aspects that are unknown and unknowable. The individuated human being that stands before us as a patient is a unique, dynamic, and multidimensional entity that is equal parts mystery and revelation. They are an impermanent, ever-changing field of paradox and complexity, influenced by their history and experience yet always capable of experiencing freedom from the tyranny of the past.

In this milieu of complexities, we seek to understand and grasp the spirit of the medicine, of the individual, of the moment. We seek to come to an experiential awareness of unity and transcendence even as we exist as embodied beings faced with the human struggle of duality—self and other, body and spirit, life and death. And yet even

---

1   This section was previously published as an article in *Acupuncture Today* (Richardson 2015).

as the body separates us, it provides us with the means to experience the physical, sensual world. Embodiment gives us the means to experience both the physical and the non-physical realities. Enlightenment, the natural state, being aligned with the *dao*...none of these are found "somewhere else." They are all accessible to us right here, right now. As it is said in Buddhist doctrine, it is through *samsara* that we find *nirvana*. In other words, it is in the physical form that the spirit becomes tangible, even as it slips away in the impermanence of each moment.

A critical understanding that is necessary to finding the balance between the art and the science of medicine is the understanding of medicine as metaphor. In a very real sense, all medical theories and perspectives are metaphors—they are metaphorical abstractions, assumptions, and generalizations about people, our environment, and the needs of the individual human. It is through such abstractions and generalizations that we are able to create models of how and why disease occurs and progresses, as well as models of what it means to be healthy. However, these models can never be exact replicas of the individual human experience. For this reason, we can say that every medical model is, in fact, a metaphor for the lived human experience of disease and health. They are necessarily limited by the fact that they are merely reference points—they are "fingers pointing to the moon;" or, as Alfred Korzybski aptly stated, "The map is not the territory." Perhaps it can be said that the closer the metaphor comes to approximating the individual's experience, the more useful it is.

It is because all medicine is metaphor that medicine is both an art and a science—we need the science of the organizing medical model, the structure of the lens through which we view each individual and imbalance, but we also need the art of knowing that each individual is unique and of choosing which lens to use in each moment. Often it is when the practitioner and patient do not consciously acknowledge the metaphorical nature of the medicine that this becomes more problematic. One of the most beautiful aspects of Chinese medicine is that it self-consciously recognizes that it is metaphorical, that it consciously draws parallels to nature, to aspects of nature that correspond to the human experience.

When we start to believe that any given model is a form of absolute truth, when we lose sight that it is only a relative perspective, the metaphor itself inevitably becomes self-limiting and therefore self-defeating. It becomes a self-limiting perspective precisely because it reifies itself, and in this way loses connection to the art of practicing medicine and seeing each patient as a unique, dynamic individual. In order to avoid such reification of perspective, it is vital to recognize that the moment-to-moment reality of the individual human experience can never be fully and adequately captured by words and models—these can never be more than approximations of the experience itself. They are merely a means of organizing and orienting the lived experience in such a way as to make meaning of the experience.

The truth of being can only be experientially realized, not told. The etymology of the word "doctor" is "to teach;" our job as practitioners of medicine is not only to help diminish patients' suffering by subjecting them to acupuncture, herbal medicine, pharmaceutical drugs, or surgery, but to help diminish their suffering through teaching them and helping them to know and understand themselves and their experience. Using the metaphorical lenses skillfully not only allows us to make a difference in our patients' experiences, but also allows us to fundamentally shift their perspective and understanding of themselves, to help them to see themselves as already whole. In this book, therefore, I present one more potential medical metaphor—one that aims to present the practice of medicine in a light not only of reducing suffering, but of encouraging and facilitating wholeness.

* * *

In the first part of this book, I set up some of the background and terminology against which this theoretical model will develop. I review concepts of Daoist cosmology, by examining the concept of the "natural state," as well as the concepts of vertical and horizontal axes of integration. I then examine some of the correspondences of the *dai mai*, one of the least often discussed of the extraordinary vessels.

In the second part of this book, I build the model. I start by following the flow of the *ying qi* through the primary channels, to examine the relationship of this cycle to the confluent points of the extraordinary vessels. In so doing, we will explore a possible connection between this cycle and a relation of the extraordinary vessels to Daoist cosmogenesis. With this foundation in place, we can then go on to explore correspondences between the extraordinary vessels and the extraordinary organs, examining the relationship of both to the cycle of the evolution of consciousness. Finally, I examine possible relationships between the extraordinary vessels and the extraordinary organs with the primary channels and *zangfu*.

❋ ❋ ❋

Unity is extraordinary. And it is the experience of such moments, the experience of something beyond the limited self, that makes life meaningful. Thank you for joining me on this journey, I hope that you may find it as extraordinary as I have!

Chapter 1

The Natural State in Daoism and Chinese Medicine

Cultivate love and compassion
And truth will prevail

Being true to oneself
The energy flows freely
And happiness ensues

Allow happiness to flourish
And love becomes the natural state
Between and among
Beings in the universe

The All requires nothing
And offers everything
This is the natural state

One of the fundamental cosmological and medical assumptions utilized throughout this book is the concept of "the natural state." This concept is present in both Daoism and Chinese medicine (as well as Buddhism), and underpins much of the Chinese medical model. In these perspectives and models, the natural state is presented as an experiential state of being in the world that is an innate potential accessible to all humans; in the natural state one is completely whole in oneself while being connected to Heaven above, Earth below, and the world around oneself. In Daoist terms, this is to be "in tune" or "aligned" with the *dao*; in Chinese medicine, this is associated with a free flow of *qi* and blood through the body. When one is in the natural state, the body has a nearly unlimited, innate capacity to heal—excesses will be carried off, and deficiencies filled, all through the smooth circulation of *qi* and blood throughout the body. In this chapter, we will examine the natural state as presented in Daoism and Chinese medical theory.[1]

The Natural State

To begin, I would first like to explore the concept of the natural state and examine some of the cognates that are used throughout the Daoist tradition; however, the tradition itself frequently maintains that any words used to describe the natural state cannot encapsulate or perfectly portray the experiential state itself. Instead, they are merely "fingers

---

1   Chinese medical philosophy and epistemology is primarily associated with Daoist and proto-Daoist cosmology and worldviews. The intent of this chapter is not to look for causation of how one aspect affected another, but to simply compare them side-by-side to flesh out similarities and differences.

pointing to the moon," rather than the moon itself—or, as the first line of the *Dao De Jing* asserts, "The *dao* that can be spoken is not the eternal *dao*." From the literature, it is clear that the terms used to describe the "natural state" refer both to the way in which one experiences oneself and the world around oneself, and to the way one acts. Besides indicating a "state" that is experienced by the human that exists as an individuated being, the terms often translated as "natural" imply that this state is something that is simultaneously innate and connected to the natural world, connected to something beyond the limited individuated being.

This dual nature of the terminology is seen in one of the Chinese character compounds that is often translated as "natural state" in the Daoist tradition, *ziran* (自然), which can literally be translated as "to be so of itself."[2] *Ziran* is often used to refer to a kind of pre-reflective spontaneity that is characteristic of one acting from the natural state; thus it carries the dual connotation of the state itself and the way in which one acts when in such a state. To be in this state and to act from this state are both referred to as being in accord with the *dao*, attaining or embodying the *dao*, or flowing with the *dao*.[3]

---

2   The pictograph *zi* (自), or self, is composed of the characters for "sun" and "moon"—thereby implying that the self is always a coming together of the polar energies of sun and moon, Heaven and Earth, and *yin* and *yang* (see Wong 1992, p. 12).

3   "The Tao is the way of heaven. It is also our original nature" (Wong 1992, p. 12). There is also a relationship here to "the uncarved block" (*pu* 樸): "Pu is a state to which we can still return if we maintain our constant de 德 or 'virtue'... 'When your constant virtue is sufficient, then you will move toward (gui 歸) a natural state (pu)'" (Allan 1997, pp. 120–121). These terms also carry a close connection to the concept of spirit, *shen* (神), in Daoist thought: "The spirit is the original nature in us" (Wong 1992, p. 35).

In Daoism, the natural state and *ziran* are closely associated with the concept of "non-action," or *wuwei* (無為):

> In the *Zhuangzi*, non-action appears as a more psychological mode and is a characteristic of spontaneity (*ziran*), the main quality of the embodied Dao. It means to be free in mind and spirit and able to wander about the world with ease and pleasure (see *yuanyou*), to engage in an ecstatic oneness with all-there-is. (*The Encyclopedia of Taoism* 2008, p. 1067)

For this reason, *ziran* is also closely associated with the terms *xiaoyao* and *yuanyou*.[4] As stated by Sarah Allan, in commenting on the *Zhuangzi*:

> [I]ntentionless movement is a common theme in [the Inner Chapters of the *Zhuangzi*]. It is most frequently expressed by the term *xiaoyao* 逍遙, often translated as "roaming" or "wandering." Thus, the sage "roams freely" or "wanders" (*xiaoyao* 逍遙) in the *dao*, just as fish swim freely in a stream... Like *wuwei*, *xiaoyao* is to be free of conscious deliberation. (1997, pp. 82–83)

This image of a fish in water indicates another important characteristic of one who is in the natural state—that they exist in a kind of non-separation with the world around them, or an "ecstatic oneness with all-there-is." As another modern commentator, Rur-Bin Yang, states:

---

4   This is also where the name for the well-known herbal formula, *xiao yao san*, or Free and Easy Wanderer, derives from.

What [this type of wandering] refers to is the emergence and circulation of the spiritual energy (*shenqi* 神氣) together with the world in a kind of super-experiential state. Its basis thus lies in the observer's elevation of himself to enter into a kind of mystical state of coexistence with the existential basis of all things. (2003, p. 113)

This is a coming together of the inner and outer worlds, of one's inner nature being in harmony with the world around oneself.

However, this can also imply that an individual is manifesting and actualizing their innate potential in the world, that they are fulfilling their destiny. As stated in *The Encyclopedia of Taoism*, "Similarly, the 'free and easy wandering'...of the *Zhuangzi* is more specifically described as the complete harmony and alignment of the human being with one's inner nature and destiny" (2008, p. 1141). When an individual exists in such a state, not only are they in harmony within and without and actualizing their destiny, they also perceive reality as it is, for they are embodying the one true reality. "*Zhuangzi* 31 defines the term saying: 'Reality (*zhen*) is what is received from Heaven; it is so of itself ([see] *ziran*) and cannot be altered (*yi* 易).' In *Zhuangzi* 2...one who has attained the Dao is called *zhenren*" (*The Encyclopedia of Taoism* 2008, p. 1265). *Zhenren* (真人) is the true or authentic person and is therefore another term that is often used to describe the individual who attains the natural state.

Along these lines, moving towards the natural state is often seen as synonymous with becoming more fully human—in other words, for the individual human being to attain the natural state is to fulfill their potential as a human. As stated by Allan, "The person who follows the *dao* is simply the most fully human" (1997, p. 68). Incidentally, this ability to follow the *dao* is closely linked to the function and development of the mind-heart (*xin* 心):

> Thus, people are not "reasoning animals" but living things which have a certain potential for growth when they are nurtured properly. As a species, they are defined by the uniqueness of their minds/hearts. Thus it is by fully developing the mind/heart that a person becomes most fully human. (Allan 1997, pp. 95–96)

Further, as noted by Wang Mu:

> A postface to *Awakening to Reality* says: "If you want to embody the supreme Dao, nothing is more important than understanding the Heart. The Heart is the axis of the Dao." According to Zhang Boduan, Heart and Spirit are related as follows: the Heart is the ultimate foundation, and Spirit is born from the Heart; the foundation of the Heart consists in non-doing and non-movement; as it moves, it is called Spirit. (2011, p. 37)

This will have important implications later on, when we turn to examine the role and relationship of the Heart to balancing above and below and the inside and the outside. To experientially exist in the natural state is thus considered the highest expression of humanity, and the highest expression of what it means to be human.

Innate Potentiality

According to the writings on the *dao* and *ziran*, the natural state is an innate potentiality that all human beings possess and have the ability to actualize. This potentiality is not about achieving or gaining something extrinsic to oneself; it is already fully present within every individual. To experientially exist in the natural state does not require movement towards something else, nor does it require one to depend on or receive anything from anyone or anything else. The natural state is something that is accessible to all of us, at all times—it is just a matter of recognizing it, and it is the shift in one's state of mind or perspective that allows one to access this potential.

In Daoism, it is understood that all individuals have the capacity to become a fully actualized and authentic person (*zhenren*); they have simply forgotten. As Eva Wong states, in commenting on the Daoist text *Cultivating Stillness*:

> Many people are ignorant and do not recognize their original nature...in reality, the Tao is not far from human existence and human existence is never far from the Tao... This means that everyone can become a sage, a buddha, or an immortal... Although your existence is in the mortal realm, your heart transcends it. (1992, pp. 24–25)[5]

---

5   This text was written no earlier than 1628 CE. Therefore, while it is primarily a Daoist text, it also clearly exhibits Buddhist influence—hence the idea that everyone can "become a sage, a Buddha, or an immortal." These three states relate to the natural state or the highest state of an adept in the *sanjiao* (三教), the three schools—in Confucianism the realized being is a sage, in Buddhism a Buddha, and in Daoism an immortal.

Not only do all people have the ability to "become a sage, a buddha, or an immortal," but the author of *Cultivating Stillness* also notes: "The sage symbolizes the goodness inherent in all sentient beings" (Wong 1992, p. 3).

As stated in *Cultivating Stillness*, "Although we speak of attaining the Tao, there is really nothing to attain" (Wong 1992, p. 89). In other words, we already have everything we need, and we do not possess anything that impedes us from being in this state. Wong elaborates on this:

> Although it is said that you attain the Tao, you are really receiving nothing at all…all the treasures described are in the body and not anywhere else. That is why it is said that you receive nothing; you possess them from the beginning. (1992, p. 90)

And as written in the *Nei-yeh* 內業 (which is believed to predate both the *Laozi* and *Zhuangzi*):

> 5 *That Way is `not distant from us;*
> 6 *When people attain it they are sustained*
> 7 *That Way is not separated from us;*
> 8 *When people accord with it they are harmonious.*

> (Cited in Roth 1999, p. 103)

In commenting on this passage, Harold Roth writes:

> These passages do not suggest that the Way is sometimes present within human beings and at other times absent. Rather, the Way is always present. However, the

awareness of this presence enters the human mind only when it is properly cultivated. (1999, p. 103)

Therefore, the only "work" to be done is the work of cultivating the ability to experientially exist in this state, to experientially realize that we already have the Way within us. Now that the Daoist foundation of the natural state has been explored, we can turn to examine its relationship to the foundations of Chinese medicine.

Chinese Medicine and the Natural State

Every system of medicine is built on an underlying cosmology and philosophy, which holds certain assumptions, beliefs, and perspectives about suffering, health, and what it means to be human; thus the concept of medicine is inherently connected to and influenced by social and cultural constructs. For this reason, there has often been an overlap and interplay—especially in their beginnings— between medical and religio-spiritual traditions. It can even be argued that in many early cultures there was not a clear division between medicine, religion, and philosophy; this is certainly true when examining the foundations of Chinese medicine, as its foundations are deeply entwined with the roots of Daoist philosophy and the conceptions of the natural state (Wong and Wu 1932).[6] In this section I

---

6   As Joseph Needham writes in "Medicine and Chinese Culture": "In China there can be little doubt that physicians (i) came from the same origin as wizards (wu). They were therefore connected with one of the deepest roots of Taoism... During the course of the ages these ['medicine-men'] differentiated into all kinds of specialized professions, not only physicians, but also Taoist alchemists, invocators

will examine the relationship between Daoist conceptions of the natural state and the perspective of Chinese medicine, by examining passages from the *Huangdi Neijing* (黃帝內經)—*The Yellow Emperor's Inner Classic.*

The *Huangdi Neijing* seamlessly interweaves discussions on cosmology, philosophy, and medical practice. As stated in the *Suwen*, "it is said that one who studies medicine must understand the knowledge of the universe—cosmology" (Ni 1995, p. 249). This text then goes on to draw direct correlations between cultivation of such knowledge and one's ability to understand the natural state. And it is through knowing the natural state that one knows what health is, and therefore one knows what disease is: "To know the natural way, one must continually cultivate one's true nature. Knowing the natural way, of course, allows one to also understand the unnatural way" (Ni 1995, p. 249). From the earliest stages of Chinese medicine, the concept of the natural state is foundational—and it is through understanding the natural state that one can then understand illness and disease (i.e. the unnatural state).

The connection between the early stages of Chinese medicine and conceptions of the natural state is fundamental to understanding the perspective and goals of Chinese medicine. The emphasis on the importance of understanding the natural state or "grasping the *dao*" is restated several times, in different ways, throughout the *Suwen's* 81 chapters:

---

and liturgiologists for the curanic religion of the Imperial court, pharmacists, veterinary leeches, priests, religious leaders, mystics and many other sorts of people. By Confucius' time...the differentiation of physicians had already fully occurred" (1966, p. 264).

I have heard that one who understands the heavens will also understand people. One who understands ancient times shall understand the present. One who has a firm grasp of energy transformations will also understand the myriad things... One who understands transformation and change will understand the essence of nature. (Ni 1995, p. 258)

Ultimately, by following the Tao and implementing its life-enhancing maxims, one can expect to live harmoniously in wellness with the ever-changing universe. (Ni 1995, p. 276)

Do not forget that the myriad things of the universe have an intimate relationship with one another. They may present as varied as yin and yang, internal and external, male and female, upper and lower, but they are all interconnected, interdependent, and intertranscendent. Let us take medicine, for example. As a medical practitioner, one should master the cosmologies of heaven and earth, understand the human mind and spirit, and grasp all sciences of nature. In this way one will have a holistic, integrated perspective, and will grasp the Tao. (Ni 1995, p. 287)[7]

---

7   It is also of note that this paragraph succinctly and directly states a theory of interdependence that is quite similar to the theory of interdependence in Buddhist philosophy. There are also many similarities in early Chinese thought to the Buddhist notion of impermanence. See Livia Kohn: "The notion of eternal change and ongoing transformation of all things, for example, is part of the very early Chinese speculation about the world. Being and non-being are alternate states of the same cycle of existence. Change is what existence means, it is neither deplorable nor delightful" (1989b, p. 202).

Therefore, while the *Neijing*'s focus is on medical practice, it is evident that to know what it means to be healthy, and thus how to understand (and treat) illness, is inseparable from how to actualize one's potential as an individual human being (i.e. by harmonizing oneself with the "ever-changing universe"). According to the text, health is primarily achieved by living in harmony and balance, both within oneself and with the environment and the world around (and above and below) oneself.

From the medical perspective, when an individual exists in such harmony they will avoid disease and live a long life:

> Thus the wise nourish life by flowing with the four seasons and adapting to cold or heat, by harmonizing joy and anger in a tranquil dwelling, by balancing yin and yang, and what is hard and soft. So it is that dissolute evil cannot reach the man of wisdom, and he will be witness to a long life. (Wu 1993, p. 39)

However, being in harmony is a complex process that involves being aware of oneself and the world around oneself, of adapting to the world even while remaining centered within oneself:

> Health and well-being can be achieved only by remaining centered with one's spirit, guarding against squandering one's energy, maintaining the constant flow of one's qi and blood, adapting to the changing seasonal and yearly macrocosmic influences, and nourishing one's self preventively. (Ni 1995, p. 265)

Here we can see several main themes of early Chinese medical thought, and the relationship they share to some of the themes of the natural state discussed above.[8] In the following sections, I will focus on the relationship of the natural state in Chinese medicine to the themes of harmony and free flow.

Harmony and Balance

The natural state is characterized by harmony and balance between oneself and the world around oneself.[9] Earlier, this balance was examined through the metaphor of a fish in water, where such harmony allows one to be in a state of non-separation with the world around oneself. It is important to emphasize that the doctrines indicate that this is a form of dynamic balance—harmony and balance do not imply a static way of being in the world or that one does not change; it is quite the contrary. In other words, to truly be in harmony and in balance means to adapt and change as the moment, the season, and the setting requires; it means a dynamic, growth-enhancing state of being, a

8   "Remaining centered with one's spirit" is presented as a key to prevention of illness, which is also an equivalent to the state of the still mind-heart: "However, if one is centered and the emotions are clear and calm, energy is abundant and resistance is strong; even when confronted with the force of the most powerful, vicious wind, one will not be invaded" (Ni 1995, p. 10).

9   This is also present in Buddhist medical philosophy. As stated in the Chinese version of the *Sutra of Golden Light* (*Jin guangming jing* 金光明經), "In accordance with the seasons of the year, the faculties and the Four Elements fluctuate between excess and depletion, causing the body to become ill. A good doctor will nurture and balance the Six Elements in accordance with the four seasons of three months each, and [give] drink, food, and medicines that are appropriate for the illness" (Salguero 2013, p. 33).

process of growing ever more fully into oneself even while simultaneously growing even more connected to the world. In Chinese medicine, the natural state is associated with the harmonization that occurs through the dynamic balance of *yin* and *yang* and their constant inter-transformation; this is the source of health and well-being. As stated in the *Suwen*:

> When yin and yang are balanced, the five zang organs function appropriately together... The key to mastering health is to regulate the yin and the yang of the body. (Ni 1995, p. 11)

> The law of yin and yang is the natural order of the universe, the foundation of all things, mother of all changes, the root of life and death. In healing, one must grasp the root of the disharmony, which is always subject to the law of yin and yang. (Ni 1995, p. 17)

This is also the foundation of all acupuncture practice. As stated in the *Lingshu*:

> So it is said, the essentials of using the needle lie in knowing how to harmonize yin and yang. In harmonizing yin and yang, the essence and qi will glow with the joining of the physical body and the qi energy... Therefore it is said, the superior doctor balances the qi. (Wu 1993, p. 30)

This emphasis on the importance of dynamic balance begins in the very first chapter of the *Neijing*; here balance is directly related to the "transformation of the energies of the universe," and thus methods to "promote energy flow" are quintessential in maintaining balance, along with meditative practices:

> In the past, people practiced the Tao, the Way of Life. They understood the principle of balance, of yin and yang, as represented by the transformation of the energies of the universe. Thus, they formulated practices such as Dao-in, an exercise combining stretching, massaging, and breathing to promote energy flow, and meditation to help maintain and harmonize themselves with the universe. (Ni 1995, p. 1)

It is by regulating and balancing the flow of *yin* and *yang* in the body and quieting the mind-heart that the spirit can remain centered and grounded within the physical space of the body, which in turn allows the sense organs to perceive clearly:

> Thus, the body of one who understands the Tao will remain strong and healthy... Those who are knowledgeable have clear orifices, perceptions, hearing, vision, smell, and taste, and are light and strong... Those who understand the principles of wholesome living tame their minds and prevent them from straying. (Ni 1995, pp. 22–23)

> Similarly, in the body, pure yang qi reaches the sensory orifices, allowing one to see, hear, smell, taste, feel, and decipher all information so that the shen/spirit can remain clear and centered. (Ni 1995, p. 17)

This relationship between harmony, perception through the sense organs, and the channels connecting the individual to the world around them is essential in understanding the Chinese medical perspective on the natural state of the individual.

Free Flow and *Xiaoyao* 逍遙

As seen above, the free flow of *qi* and blood in the channels is closely related to harmony and balance within the individual, and is a significant factor affecting health and disease prevention in the *Huangdi Neijing*. In other words, when one is in harmony and balance within oneself and with the world, then the *qi* and blood flow freely through the channels, and vice versa—if the *qi* and blood flow freely, then the individual will be in a state of harmony and balance. In terms of physical aspects of health, it is a lack in the free flow of *qi* and blood that is said to give rise to all disease. As stated in the *Suwen*: "All disorders can be attributed to the blood and qi not arriving at certain streams and valleys and caves [i.e. acupuncture points]" (Ni 1995, p. 43) and "Regardless of the type of illness, one must first regulate and balance the flow of qi and blood" (Ni 1995, p. 84).[10]

---

10 Harper sums this up nicely: "By the second century BC, the vessels (*mai* 脈) carrying blood (*xue* 血) and vapour (*qi* 氣) through the body were seen to constitute the essential physiological structure around which the other constituents of the body were organized. The ascendancy of vessel theory was spurred by a still new, universal model of illness that attributed illness (or nameable ailments) to dysfunctions within the system of vessels. In contrast to older ideas that ailments were the consequence of demonic agents or pathogens occupying the patient's body, the new model considered an ailment to be the manifestation of a deeper physiological dysfunction. The goal of diagnosis and treatment was to determine the nature of the dysfunction and to re-establish somatic harmony... Vessel theory provided a framework for the application of yinyang 陰陽 and Five Agent (wuxing 五行) theories to the human organism" (2001, p. 99).

This free flow of *qi* through the vessels is directly related to the "free and easy wandering" (*xiaoyao* or *yuanyou*) of the individual in the natural state; when the channels are open and the *qi* and blood are flowing freely, the individual is thereby able to enter into the state of complete connection and non-separation with the world around them—just as a fish in water. As stated by a modern commentator examining this process in the Daoist tradition:

> Once the entire body is transformed by the vital energy—that is, when the adept's body has become manifest to the full—the sense organs and body that had originally been used to support or restrain one into individuality have now become, on the contrary, the channels through which the individual flows into and interconnects with the outer world. (Yang 2003, p. 110)

This process of interconnection can also be seen as a process of "reconnection," whereby the individual returns to the primordial oneness that is the natural state of humanity within this perspective. As stated by Kohn:

> The One is divided into the two forces yin and yang, and they are its functions. However, in the course of their interaction in the world, the two forces establish a harmony. Thus there are three, the third being a newly found, recovered unity on the basis of the One that was divided originally. The number three consequently implies a totality as complete as was the original unity of the One. Three is a oneness on a more complex level... The notion is then associated with other classical sets of three, such as the three main agents of the universe—

heaven, earth, and humanity (Baopuzi 18). (1989a, pp. 129–130)

In Chinese cosmology, one corresponds to Heaven, two corresponds to Earth, and three corresponds to Humanity—thus the individual human is the "newly found, recovered unity on the basis of the One that was divided originally." Humans are the coming together of Heaven above and Earth below, and the channels are the flow of *qi* connecting these two polarities to create the bipolar unity of the human being, which then becomes "oneness on a more complex level."

In accordance with Chinese cosmology, this flow of *qi* has a direct relationship to Heaven above and Earth below, as seen in the *Suwen*: "The most important element in clinical diagnosis is to know the relationships between heaven, earth, and humankind... The qi of the body flows in accordance with the changes of heaven and earth" (Ni 1995, p. 58). It is this free flow in the channels that connects Heaven and Earth within the individuated human and balances the flow and transformation of *yin* and *yang* within the body: "People's qi circulates ceaselessly, similar to the constantly regenerating quality of nature... The blood and qi within the body circulate throughout the channels and vessels, balancing yin and yang, just as water in rivers and lakes circulates endlessly" (Ni 1995, p. 194).[11] However, the flow of *qi* regulates not only the *yin* and *yang* of above and below (Heaven and Earth) but also

---

11   Also see Vivienne Lo: "A regulated flow of qi, the vital substance of life, was as basic to physical health as it was to the harmony of heaven and earth, and the channels through which it flowed were as carefully mapped as the waterways of the empire" (2001, p. 31).

the relationship of inside and outside: "So you have one yin and one yang. The qi of the yin and of the yang move unobstructed throughout the entire body. This is because of the interplay of the yin and yang and the relationship of the exterior and interior" (Ni 1995, p. 29).

An interesting difference that can be noted here is that the emphasis on free flow and harmony in the *Neijing* is focused on the free flow of *qi* and blood within the 12 primary channels as well as the *zangfu*; in many Daoist texts the emphasis tends to be more on free flow and harmony between the three *dantian*. The 12 primary channels and *zangfu* are associated more with the physical and mundane aspects of life (eating, breathing, sleeping, eliminating, etc.), whereas the three *dantian* are more associated with spiritual transformation. Both traditions, however, emphasize the importance of free flow between the individual and the environment, and above and below.

The emphasis on the three *dantian* in Daoism can easily be seen through two of the foundational meditation practices within this tradition—internal alchemy and the microcosmic orbit. In the practice of internal alchemy, the intention is to transform *jing* into *qi*, and *qi* into *shen* to connect with the *dao*; this is a vertical movement up the central channel from the lower to middle to upper *dantian*. In the microcosmic orbit meditation, the practitioner guides the *qi* up the *du mai* and down the *ren mai*; the intention of this practice is to balance *yin* (*ren mai*) and *yang* (*du mai*) as well as front and back, side to side, and the three *dantian*. The relationship between these different aspects of focus in Daoism and Chinese medicine will be of importance in the following chapters, and relates to the difference between the mundane and the spiritual perspectives, between the vertical and horizontal axes of integration, and between the primary channels and extraordinary vessels.

Through these ideas of harmony and balance between *yin* and *yang*, and free flow in the channels, it is possible to construct a generalized picture of the natural state of health and humanity according to Daoist texts and the *Huangdi Neijing*. In highly simplistic terms, this can be stated as the coming together, interpenetration, and harmony of the *yin* and *yang* aspects of being (Heaven and Earth, body and spirit, and inside and outside) in the individuated human, which occurs when there is free flow of *qi* and blood in the channels. This, then, gives us a view of the individual as a bipolar unity, composed of physical and non-physical aspects, that is simultaneously separate from and yet always connected to the world around oneself. Taking into account both perspectives, and their similarities and differences, can engender a deeper understanding of the nuances of the natural state and what it means to be human, and will prepare us to examine the relationship of the primary channels and extraordinary vessels in impeding or aiding the individual in attaining this state.

Chapter 2

VERTICAL AND HORIZONTAL INTEGRATION

The Dynamic Flow of Qi at the Level of Humanity

In the last chapter, I reviewed Daoist cosmological concepts and their relationship to Chinese medical theory and practice, particularly in relationship to the natural state. As seen in that discussion, one of the primary characteristics of the natural state is the seamless interpenetration of *yin* and *yang*, as represented in the individual human by the coming together of Heaven and Earth, and the inside and the outside. Throughout this book I will refer to these two different vectors of interpenetration of *yin* and *yang* as the vertical (Heaven and Earth) and horizontal (inside and outside) axes of connection and integration. This concept of humanity as a coming together and pivot of the vertical and horizontal axes of *yin* and *yang* has a direct relationship to the evolution of consciousness, and is one means of exploring and understanding humanity's place within the cosmos—as well as elucidating the natural state and what it means to be human. This chapter explores the concepts of vertical and horizontal integration and some of the ways they are expressed in the theory and practice of Chinese medicine; later chapters will continue to build upon this perspective.

In Chapter 42 of the *Dao De Jing* it is written that:

> *The Dao gives birth to one*
> *The one gives birth to two*
> *The two gives birth to three*
> *The three gives birth to the ten thousand things*
>
> *The ten thousand things carry yin and embrace yang*
> *They mix these things to embrace harmony*

Here we can see the fundamental underpinnings of Daoist cosmogenesis—in the beginning is only *dao*, which then gives birth to one (which corresponds to the *wuji* (無極), and also represents Heaven), which gives birth to two (which corresponds to the *taiji* (太极), or great polarity, and also represents Heaven and Earth), which gives birth to three (Heaven, Earth, and Humanity), which then gives birth to the ten thousand things (which refers to everything manifest at the level of humanity). As each of the ten thousand things become manifest at the level of humanity, they achieve harmony (or the natural state) through the fluid interpenetration of *yin* and *yang*, and in this manner attain "oneness on a more complex level." This is a process of each individuated being connecting body and spirit within oneself (vertical integration), and thereafter connecting the inside and the outside by connecting with all else that is present at the level of humanity (horizontal integration). Through this process, eventually there occurs the dissolution of boundaries and a return to oneness to start the process over again; this happens at both micro and macro levels throughout the individual lifetime and the universe as a whole. Thus, at death, the body and spirit separate and the body returns to Earth while the spirit ascends to Heaven.

When the *dao* splits into Heaven and Earth, it creates a polarity of *yin* and *yang*. The nature of polarity is that it is comprised of two seemingly oppositional aspects which are in relationship to each other, and therefore still part of one whole. If they were not in relationship to each other, and were instead two completely separate entities, there would be no polarity. And every time there is a polarity, there is something that simultaneously connects and separates the two polar aspects, and thus offers the opportunity to transcend and include the polar aspects to create a bipolar unity—this corresponds to the number three. In Daoist cosmology, Humanity is the pivot that simultaneously connects and separates the polar aspects of *yin* and *yang*, Earth and Heaven, and inside and outside. Being found between Heaven and Earth, Humanity is often referred to as the Middle Kingdom.[1] Every individuated being that exists at the level of humanity is thus a conduit for connecting the *qi* of *yin* and *yang*; this maintains the unity between the two polar aspects, and allows each individuated being to be a microcosmic reflection of the original Oneness. This process of vertical and horizontal integration corresponds

---

1   This is reflected in China's name: *Zhong Guo* (literally, "Middle Kingdom").

to the dynamic flow of *qi* and is one aspect in the evolution of consciousness.[2] In the natural state, these aspects of *yin* and *yang* make contact and integrate in a dynamic process of transformation and growth.

If the level of humanity is seen as a coming together of above and below and the inside and the outside, then these two axes create pivots upon which each individual being experiences and practices the art of humanity—the art of moving towards the natural state. It is through the dynamic integration of these *yin* and *yang* aspects of being that one is able to have a direct experience of being human, of being incarnated at this level. As seen in Chapter 1, in the natural state the *qi* flows smoothly within the body, without blockage, as well as through the body—*qi* from Heaven flowing down through the individual and into Earth, and *qi* from Earth flowing up through the body to Heaven. In this state, not only does the individual have a nearly unlimited, innate capacity to heal physically, emotionally, mentally, and spiritually, but they also exist in a state of experiential awareness—simultaneously experiencing the interconnectedness to the primordial, original oneness even as they exist at the level of duality.

Three *Dantian* and Five *Zangfu*

The vertical and horizontal axes are reflected in many aspects of Chinese medicine. At one level, the vertical axis is

---

2   A more macro view leads us to a *yin-yang* dynamic of space and time. Within the space-time dynamic, the vertical and horizontal axes are a subdivision of space: "The subdividing of space vertically and horizontally is a *yin-yang* division of *yin*" (Morris 2009; personal communication).

mirrored by the three *dantian*, while the horizontal axis is mirrored by the *zangfu*. Within the microcosm of the human body, the lower *dantian* is each individual's internal reflection of the macrocosmic Earth, while the upper *dantian* is the internal reflection of the macrocosmic Heaven. In the theory of Chinese medicine, this is seen in the way in which the three *yin* meridians of the legs (Spleen, Liver, and Kidney) all start at the feet and bring *yin qi* from the Earth up through the legs to fill the lower *dantian*, while the *yang* meridians of the arms (Large Intestine, San Jiao, and Small Intestine) all start at the fingertips and bring *yang qi* from Heaven to the face and head to fill the upper *dantian*.

Just as the individual human is a coming together of Heaven above and Earth below, in the paradigm of the three *dantian* the Heavenly *qi* of the upper *dantian* meets the Earthly *qi* of the lower *dantian* in the middle *dantian*, which is our own internal reflection of the macrocosmic level of humanity. In the Daoist tradition, this occurs along the vertical axis that runs through the center of the body from *huiyin* REN-1 to *baihui* DU-20, connecting the three *dantian*. This axis is often referred to as the *taiji* pole, and is also known as the *zhong mai* (Central Channel) or as a branch of the *chong mai* (Penetrating Vessel), one of the extraordinary vessels.

Once the Heavenly/*yang qi* of the upper *dantian* meets with the Earthly/*yin qi* of the lower *dantian* in the middle *dantian*, it is able to expand out from the central, vertical axis to connect to the rest of humanity. This unified *qi* flows out through the shoulders, arms and hands to connect with everything else present at the level of humanity— as humans we wave to each other, shake and hold hands, hug and embrace, and touch—all means of sharing *qi* and connecting with others at the level of humanity. Thus, in *qigong* practice, *baihui* DU-20 is the point that exchanges *qi* with Heaven, *yongquan* K-1 receives and exchanges *qi* with Earth, and *laogong* PC-8 (in the center of the palm) is the point that exchanges *qi* with others at the level of humanity. This expansion outward from (and return to) the central axis is representative of the horizontal axis, and is more associated with the five *zangfu* organs (which represent the four lateral directions and the center).

We can further explore the concepts of vertical and horizontal integration through examination of the character etymology of the word "King/Emperor" (*wáng* 王).[3] This character is composed of three horizontal lines connected by one central vertical line. As seen previously, one horizontal line (一) is the number "one" and also represents Heaven. Two horizontal lines (二) is the number "two" and represents Heaven and Earth. Three horizontal lines (三) is the number "three" and represents the trinity of Heaven, Earth, and Humanity. The character "Emperor/King" (王) is composed of these three horizontal lines connected by a vertical line, as the Emperor was the one who connected Heaven, Earth, and all of Humanity.

Within the microcosm of the human body, this may explain why the Heart is often called the "Emperor" among the *zangfu* organs. The Heart resides at the level of middle *dantian*, and is responsible for connecting our internal reflection of Heaven (upper *dantian*) and Earth (lower *dantian*) with all of Humanity. The Heart is, therefore, the primary organ responsible for maintaining the balance between vertical and horizontal integration of the *yin* and

---

3   This discussion is drawn from Harbaugh 1999.

yang aspects of being, connecting the three *dantian* and the inside and the outside. Perhaps it is for this reason that Daoist texts emphasize the importance of the heart/mind (*xin*) in attaining the natural state. As the Heart is a microcosmic reflection of the macrocosmic human, each individual being thus has the capacity to become an "emperor" through the processes of vertical and horizontal integration.

This correspondence between the three *dantian* and the vertical axis, and the *zangfu* organs with the horizontal axis, is seen throughout Daoist literature; the Heart is at the center (and meeting point) of both of these axes. As stated by Fabrizio Pregadio (2015):

> The heart (*xin*) is the symbolic center of the human being... But just like Unity takes multiple forms in the cosmos, so does the center of the human being reappear in multiple locations. The most important ones are the three Cinnabar Fields (*dantian*, immaterial loci in the regions of the brain, the heart, and the abdomen) and the five viscera (*wuzang*, namely liver, heart, spleen, lungs, and kidneys). The three Cinnabar Fields and the five viscera represent, respectively, the vertical and horizontal dimensions of the cosmos within the human being.

And by Isabelle Robinet: "Shangqing cosmology follows the traditional Chinese pattern based on the numbers 3 and 5...: a vertical threefold division into Heaven, Earth, and Humanity corresponds to a horizontal fivefold division into the wuxing" (*The Encyclopedia of Taoism* 2008, p. 864). The three *dantian* therefore correspond primarily to the vertical axis, and the five *zangfu* to the horizontal axis. As we will see throughout this chapter, as well as throughout the rest of this book, these axes are also seen in the pulses, the dynamic flow of *qi* (ascending–descending, entering–exiting), the Fire element, the extraordinary vessels and *fu*, and the concepts of pre- and post-heaven.

Pre- and Post-Heaven

It can be said that vertical integration corresponds to pre-heaven, while horizontal integration corresponds to post-heaven.[4] Pre-heaven, in a broad sense, relates to the individual's connection to Source, to the deep, constitutional aspects of being, the place that one comes from, and the place one returns to when one needs to center and ground within self. These characteristics of pre-heaven are also reflected by the extraordinary vessels, which, within the channel systems, correspond relatively more to pre-heaven and the Source. As stated by Claude Larre and Elisabeth Rochat de la Vallée:

> The meaning is that because these meridians are older, more ancient than the ordinary meridians, when extraordinary circumstances exist outside, and the twelve main meridians can no longer ensure the

---

4   It should be noted that throughout this book I use pre-heaven and post-heaven very broadly—that they relate not only to chronological periods of time in one's life (before and after birth) or forms of *jing* (congenital and acquired), but to an ongoing interplay between the individual's Source/essence (and what they are here for), and the way they begin to manifest that in the world (as well as the way in which their experience in the world impacts the individual).

maintenance of the twelve areas of the body, there is a return to a more ancient and deeper regulation of life. (1997, p. 11)

Thus, the extraordinary vessels (which correspond to pre-heaven) are also what one returns to in order to center and ground within self during extraordinary times.

Post-heaven, on the other hand, is that which is experienced at the horizontal level, connecting with everything else in one's environment. Therefore, post-heaven is often associated with the digestive system and *wei qi*, the means of processing, interacting with, and integrating that which is experienced at the human level of reality. For these reasons, while the extraordinary vessels and organs as a whole may be considered to correspond to pre-heaven, the primary channels correspond more to post-heaven—they are the channels that work more with the daily functions of life, of breathing, eating, interacting with others, and so forth—and thus correspond more to horizontal integration and processing interactions with the world around oneself.

This relationship between pre-heaven and post-heaven also has a relationship to conceptions of the evolution of consciousness—from the Source or lower *dantian* (pre-heaven), the *qi* expands outward, leading to creation, manifestation, and integration within oneself, the creation of the channels, *zangfu*, and the sense organs. From this movement of expansion from the Source outwards, the primary meridians, *zangfu*, and sense organs are then the means by which one experiences the exterior world (post-heaven), which, in experiencing it, also guides it back to pre-heaven to be integrated and processed (thus producing *qi* and essence, replenishing the Source, impacting/ transforming one at the deepest level, and allowing one to start the cycle over again).

The Dynamic Flow of *Qi*

The axes of vertical and horizontal integration are likely related to what has been referred to in the classics as the "ascending and descending of *qi*" (vertical) and "entering and exiting of *qi*" (horizontal). The collective ascending– descending and entering–exiting of *qi* is also what has been translated by some as the "*qi* mechanism" or the "*qi* dynamic." In this section, excepting direct citations, I will refer to this as the "dynamic flow of *qi*" to emphasize the fluidity of this process.

In Chapter 68 of the *Su Wen* (Simple Questions) it is stated:

> If there is no ascending/descending, there is no birth, growth, maturation and decline. If there is no entering/ exiting, there is no birth, growth, transformation, receiving and storage. If the Qi Mechanism functions well there is room for birth and transformation; if the Qi Mechanism is disrupted, there is fragmentation and no birth or transformation. (Cited in Maciocia 2005, p. 78)

As this passage is central to the discussion, it is worthwhile to look at another translation:

> Thus, if there is no going out and coming in, there will be no process of birth, growth, robustness, senility and

death; if there is no ascent and descent, there will be no process of generating, growth, blooming, yielding fruit or crop and finally storing. So, in all visible things, they are having the energies of going out, coming in, ascent and descent. Therefore the existence of growth and transformation depends upon the existence of the visible things. If the visible body disappeared, the growth and transformation will be extinguished. So, none of the visible things are without the energies of going out, coming in, ascent and descent, only there are the differences in extent and the earlier or later in time. (Wang 1997, p. 336)

It is interesting to note that this translation states that all "visible things" (which are the ten thousand things present at the level of humanity) have this dynamic flow of *qi* occurring, and, further, that all growth/generation and transformation depends on the visible things.

It is through harmony in this process of the ascending–descending, entering–exiting of *qi* that one is able to achieve a state of health, happiness, and freedom—which is synonymous with the natural state, the state of experiential awareness. As seen in the quotation above, without vertical integration (ascending/descending) and horizontal integration (entering/exiting), life is not possible. Life itself is the process of connecting above and below and the inside and the outside; without this continuous exchange, it is not possible for one to continue at this level of existence. Vertical integration allows for maturation and decline, as it is the connection to Source and related to our path and fundamental purpose here on Earth; horizontal integration is what allows for transformation, receiving, and storage, as it relates to post-heaven, digestion, and the connection to everything else at the level of humanity. It is experiencing and interacting with that which is around and inside oneself that allows an individual to transform.

These axes are reflected at every level throughout the body, from the macro to the micro.

> The ascending–descending and entering–exiting of Qi influences the formation of Qi and Blood at every stage and in every organ. The very production of Qi and Blood relies on the delicate, harmonious balance of ascending–descending and entering–exiting of Qi in every organ, every part of the body, every structure and at every stage. (Maciocia 2005, p. 78)

The dynamic flow of *qi* also relates to the ability to sense (and therefore experience) clearly, as stated by Zhou Xue Hai in "Notes on Reading Medical Books": "The faculties of seeing, hearing, smelling, tasting and thinking all depend on the smooth ascending/descending and entering/exiting of Qi; if Qi is obstructed [in its ascending/descending and entering/exiting] those faculties are not normal" (cited in Maciocia 2005, p. 78). Thus, from the macro to the micro level, the vertical and horizontal axes are an integral part of the individual's experience not only to live, but to experience life at the most intricate levels.

The Fire Element

We can also see the axes of vertical and horizontal integration represented within the Fire element. Fire is what transforms and connects across boundaries, and is therefore the element responsible for the connection and transformation across both the vertical and horizontal axes—just as the Heart (which pertains to Fire) is at the center of both axes and balances between them. This may be seen in the properties of Fire—not only does it flare upward (vertically), but it also expands laterally (horizontally). Looking at it from this perspective, we can readily find support in the literature for the two different forms of Fire—vertical, as represented by the Emperor Fire, and horizontal, as represented by the Ministerial Fire. As stated by Giovanni Maciocia, "Thus, purely from a Five-Element perspective, the Pericardium pertains to the Minister Fire (with the Triple Burner) compared to the Emperor Fire of the Heart" (2005, p. 167).

There are two pairs of *zangfu* organs associated with the Fire element—the Heart–Small Intestine and the Pericardium–San Jiao. The Heart is well known to be the Emperor, as it connects Heaven, Earth, and Humanity, as seen above. Similarly, the Small Intestine is the "middle" connection in the digestive system, connecting the Stomach above with the Large Intestine below, and may thus be seen as the "emperor" within the digestive system. Therefore, it is the Emperor Fire of the Heart and Small Intestine that regulates vertical integration, the connection between above and below at both micro and macro levels.

On the other hand, the Pericardium (*xinbao*) and San Jiao are referred to as the Ministers, and are the *zangfu* that connect the emperor with its subjects and the rest of the kingdom (horizontal integration). The Pericardium is the wrapping of the Heart, a boundary that simultaneously connects the Heart to (and separates it from) the rest of the "kingdom" (i.e. the other *zangfu* and the exterior).

Similarly, the San Jiao is often depicted as the three body cavities—the boundaries that simultaneously connect and separate the *zangfu* from the rest of the body and the exterior. Thus the Ministerial Fire, as the Pericardium and San Jiao, relates relatively more to horizontal integration—connecting one with everything else present at the level of humanity.

When it is in balance, the Emperor Fire stays in the Heart—maintaining the vertical connection within self, between Heaven, Earth, Humanity—while it is the Ministerial Fire that goes out to connect. It is the Ministerial Fire that descends from the Heart to the Kidneys, and is associated with the Kidney Yang and *mingmen*. For this reason, both the Pericardium–San Jiao and Kidney Yang–*mingmen* are all referred to as the Ministerial Fire, and relate to the desire for intimacy and connection with everything else present at the level of humanity. Interestingly, *mingmen* is often translated as "Gate of Life." It is only through this horizontal connection of the Ministerial Fire that one can be born, transform, and live. Further, there is an interesting parallel in the term "Gate," as a gate is a boundary that opens and closes, and it is only through this form of exchange across boundaries opening and closing that life occurs. Similarly, the Pericardium and San Jiao, when in balance, open and close at the appropriate times, thereby regulating what (or who) is allowed into our selves and our hearts.

In the pulse, all of these aspects have been said to correspond to the right proximal position according to various systems; this position is also sometimes associated with the reproductive and circulatory systems, both of which may also be seen primarily as aspects of the Ministerial Fire.

The drive to reproduce is the desire to connect intimately with another, to become "one" with another, and thus is a fundamental aspect of horizontal integration. Reproduction itself is the birthing of a new being at the horizontal/ human level of reality. Likewise, the circulatory system is the means of communication and connection between the Emperor (Heart) and the rest of the kingdom.

Continuing, we can see that the vertical and horizontal axes are well reflected in several aspects of the pulse. While each of the pulse positions (*cun, guan,* and *chi*) on each side has its own organ correspondences, each side as a whole is often used to represent certain systemic patterns relating to the fundamental polarity of *yin* and *yang* as it manifests throughout the body. If we apply this to the ideas of vertical and horizontal integration, it becomes clear that the left-hand pulse corresponds to the vertical axis, while the right-hand pulse corresponds to the horizontal axis.

In general, the left-hand pulse (Heart–Liver–Kidney) is said to correspond to the *yin* aspects of being (including blood, essence, *yuan qi,* and pre-heaven) and the right-hand pulse (Lung–Spleen–Pericardium) to the *yang* aspects of being (*qi,* digestion, *wei qi,* post-heaven).[5] If the left-hand pulse corresponds to pre-heaven, then it can also correspond to vertical integration, as seen above. This is reinforced by the fact that the Liver connects the Fire of the Heart with the Water of the Kidneys in the generating cycle, creating

---

5   The perspective of the left-hand pulse corresponding to pre-heaven and the right-hand pulse to post-heaven comes from Neoclassical Pulse Diagnosis as an interpretation from the Shen-Hammer system of pulse diagnosis (Morris, personal communication). The vertical and horizontal axes are also represented within the Neoclassical system in the Compass Model (see Morris 2002a).

the axis of vertical integration within the *zangfu* organs.[6] Similarly, the Lung–Spleen–Pericardium axis corresponds to post-heaven, the production of *wei qi*, and the digestive system; all of these aspects are representative of the horizontal axis.

Continuing the above discussion on the Fire element in regard to the pulse, it is clear that both aspects of the Fire element are well placed to reflect their associations. The left distal position belongs to the Heart and Small Intestine, and thus corresponds to the Emperor Fire—and again, the left-hand pulse and the Emperor Fire both correspond to vertical integration. The right proximal position, as seen above, is said to relate to Kidney Yang–*mingmen*, Pericardium–San Jiao, or circulatory–reproductive systems, all of which also fall under the category of Ministerial Fire—and it is the right-hand pulse and the Ministerial Fire that correspond to horizontal integration. Thus, the right proximal position, the Ministerial Fire, is the root of post-heaven, of the digestive processes as well as *wei qi*, and therefore the root of (as well as the impetus towards) horizontal integration. And the left distal position, the Emperor Fire, is the fruition of each individual connecting Heaven and Earth, of vertical integration and the connection with self and to Source.

---

6   "The wood element is located between water and fire along the *sheng* cycle. A function of the wood element is to regulate the smooth flow of *qi* between fire and water just as the *chongqi* must harmonize the dual poles of heaven and earth. Physiologically, the liver and gallbladder that regulate *qi* are located in the middle heater, and the jing stored in the kidneys and the *shen* stored in the heart are located in the lower and upper heater, respectively... It is the liver's virtue of benevolence (*ren*) that allows *shen* and *jing* to interact in an unconstrained manner" (Jarrett 2004, pp. 236–237).

Dynamic Balance

Qi is dynamic; in the natural state *qi* is constantly flowing throughout one's being. *Qi* is never static unless it is pathological; experiential awareness is simply the art of experiencing the dynamic flow of *qi*. Vertical integration is a process of *qi* coming in and integrating within oneself, and horizontal integration is that of the exchange and unification between the inside and the outside. Dynamic balance between vertical and horizontal integration allows for continuous cycles of growth, connection to Source, and the evolution of consciousness—as they balance, each can continually grow, and as they evolve, so does the individual.

When speaking of horizontal integration, vertical integration is already presupposed. The horizontal integration depends on, and always refers back to, vertical integration. It is similar to discussing post-heaven—whenever one discusses post-heaven, it automatically refers back to pre-heaven, as post-heaven cannot exist without pre-heaven and is dependent on a continuous integration with pre-heaven. Pre-heaven is the blueprint, just as vertical integration is the foundation. It is only by having the vertical integration of *jing* and *shen*, Body and Spirit, that one can then experience horizontal connection and integration.

As the vertical connection grows stronger, one eventually needs to extend out and connect with others at the level of humanity. As the horizontal connection grows, the vertical connection may diminish and thus one needs to come back to center and strengthen it. If the vertical connection diminishes, one may be more easily affected by everything else in one's environment, for they are less rooted in themselves and the Source. This balancing between vertical and horizontal is similar to balancing between masculine and feminine, Body and Spirit, and *yin* and *yang*—in order for both to grow there must be a dynamic balance between them, so that they might continuously generate and transform each other. By returning to the vertical connection and dynamically integrating the vertical and horizontal axes, one enters a state of experiential awareness and can freely experience the level of humanity.

Vertical integration allows one to be firmly rooted in the essence, so that awareness may grow and one may experience more at the horizontal level. As one becomes more whole and integrated within oneself (connected to Heaven and yet rooted in Earth), one is able to be open to and connect with everything and everyone else. This can occur in degrees and cycles at both micro and macro levels; it is a process of learning to stay true to oneself while simultaneously experiencing the external and internal environments. This allows one to connect with others externally while staying centered within, and thus attain greater degrees of experiential awareness of both the internal and external worlds. Therefore, although the axes are each representative of a polarity or pivot (Heaven–Earth, Interior–Exterior), they themselves form a *yin–yang* (vertical–horizontal) polarity that corresponds to the dynamic flow of *qi*. And, as with all polarities, the key to growth, freedom, and happiness—to attaining the natural state—is dynamic balance and free flow.

Chapter 3

THE *DAI MAI*

*Dynamic Structural Flexibility
and Spherical Integration*

Now that we have reviewed some of the pertinent concepts within Daoist cosmology and Chinese medical theory, we can turn our view towards the extraordinary vessels. Perhaps one of the most fascinating aspects that arises when one begins to investigate the extraordinary vessels is that although they are said to relate to the deep, constitutional level of being, their understanding and use seems to remain relatively peripheral in the contemporary practice of Traditional Chinese Medicine. Starting from the lower *dantian*, they are considered to be the source of all creation, yet these vessels lack any form of solid theory integrating them with the primary channel and *zangfu* organ systems. Among the extraordinary vessels, the *dai mai*, or Girdling Vessel, often seems to be one of the least understood.

In this chapter I examine some of the correspondences and associations of the *dai mai* in an attempt to gain a greater understanding of the sphere of energetic function of this extraordinary vessel and its relation to the *zangfu* organs and primary channels. This perspective is primarily based on examining its relation to the dynamic flow of *qi* at the level of humanity. After exploring the importance of the *dai mai*, we can then turn to examining the relationship of the extraordinary vessels as a whole to Daoist conceptions of the evolution of consciousness.

As discussed in the last chapter, the level of humanity is often referred to as the Middle Kingdom, or *zhong guo*. The first character, *zhong* (中, middle), is written contemporarily as a square bifurcated by a vertical line. This character, which is translated as middle or center, may provide insight into the cosmological place of humanity as the "middle," and its relation to the dynamic flow of *qi*. Historically, the character was written similarly, except it was a circle— instead of a square—encompassing the vertical straight line. If we return to the idea that humans connect Heaven above and Earth below, then it is likely that the vertical line represents this central connection of vertical integration.

This is seen in the *zhong* (中) *mai*, or central channel, which travels from *huiyin* REN-1 to *baihui* DU-20 through the center of the body and connects the three *dantian* (our own internal reflections of the macrocosmic Heaven, Earth, and Humanity). Similarly, one could look at the flow of the primary meridians, flowing from the tips of the fingers (stretching up towards Heaven) down to the tips of the toes (reaching down into Earth) and vice versa, creating a flow of *qi* between Heaven and Earth. What then of the square (or circle) through which this central channel of energy passes? It seems quite plausible that if this character corresponds to the dynamic flow of *qi* at the level of humanity, then the circle can be seen as corresponding to the level of horizontal integration, as well as the *dai mai*. According to Li Zhong Zi, "Dai mai is like an horizontal link tying together all the network of animation, all the circulation, and it corresponds to the six junctions, liu he (六合)" (cited in Larre and Rochat de la Vallée 1997, pp. 18–19). The *dai mai* is the one meridian that travels horizontally around the body, and is responsible for binding and connecting all of the vertically traveling meridians, and thus corresponds to the six junctions—the four cardinal directions with above and below.

The *dai mai*, in binding all of the vertically flowing energy, may play a central role in holding humanity at this "middle" level between Heaven and Earth by providing a structure/container for the *qi* so that it does not simply dissipate. Without something binding all of the vertically flowing *qi*, it seems likely that everything would disperse, and the physical body would disintegrate back into the Earth and the spirit would ascend into Heaven; perhaps within the extraordinary vessels, it is the *dai mai* that performs this function and keeps us present at this level. At the level of humanity there is a coming together of body and spirit; I suggest that the *dai mai* assists in this vertical integration of body and spirit by providing dynamic structural flexibility.

Dynamic structural flexibility refers to the energetic aspect that regulates contraction and expansion of an individual's boundaries in relation to their environment. It allows the *qi* to flow freely, allowing for a more complete integration of body and spirit at this level, even as one interacts with everything else present at the level of humanity. The *dai mai* creates a boundary at the horizontal level of integration, a boundary that simultaneously connects one to and separates one from everything else present at the level of humanity, and in this way may provide the function of dynamic structural flexibility at this level.

The Wood Element

The *dai mai*, in binding all of the vertically flowing meridians, has a major impact on astringing/tightening (as well as dispersing/slackening) at the horizontal level and, in so doing, affects/directs the energy towards vertical integration. If humans connect Heaven and Earth, and it is when the *qi* flows smoothly through the body that one is happy and healthy, what better example is there for us at the level of humanity than the tree? A tree reaches its roots deep into the Earth as its branches stretch up into Heaven, thus connecting above and below and allowing the *qi* to flow smoothly between Heaven and Earth.

In looking at a tree, the trunk is composed of rings, which are reminiscent of the *zhong* character and the *dai mai*. Just as the trunks of trees are cylindrical, which (by astringing and providing circular integrity) allows the qi to flow primarily between Heaven and Earth, so too may the *dai mai* function similarly for humans. As stated by Larre and Rochat de la Vallée:

> [The *dai mai*] is able to ensure the binding, but with a kind of relaxation. If it is too relaxed there is erratic circulation, congestion and knots. If it is too tight there may be other kinds of blockage and congestion. It must be able to keep a good balance between what is going down and what is coming up. (1997, p. 149)

The size of the rings of a tree vary depending on the external conditions, which indicates that there is also a correlation between the size of the ring and the amount that the tree is exchanging/connecting with the external environment at that point in time. Wood grows vertically, but also horizontally—perhaps it is the circular integrity and dynamic structural flexibility provided by the *dai mai* that balances these two vectors of growth and exchange within the individuated human.

Within the human body, the Wood element is primarily associated with the Liver and Gall Bladder. Here too we can see that Wood is closely associated with the process of vertical integration as it is the Liver that connects the Water of the Kidneys with the Fire of the Heart in the generating cycle, as discussed in the previous chapter. Sinews and tendons pertain to Wood, and are responsible for maintaining the balance between flexibility and structure— that is, maintaining a flexible structure for optimal growth and connection between above and below and the inside and the outside; a structure that is stable enough to house the spirit and yet flexible enough to still allow it the freedom to flourish. This is also reflected in the properties of Wood: bamboo is often used in Oriental culture and medicine as a stunning example of the importance of flexibility to achieve growth. If it was not flexible enough to bend with the wind, it would break, and yet as soon as the wind stops blowing the bamboo returns upright to continue growing towards Heaven. This shows the strength to remain true to its course while remaining flexible enough to adapt to moment-to-moment obstacles that may arise.

Zulinqi GB-41, confluent point of the *dai mai*, is located on the border of a tendon and is the Wood point of the Gall Bladder channel; this further indicates a close association between the *dai mai*, the Wood element, and the tendons, and how they share this function of balancing flexibility and structure. When one has excessive tension, it impedes one's ability to experience; similarly, if one lacks proper tension/boundaries that will also impede one's ability to stay true to oneself and thus diminish one's capacity for experiential awareness. Therefore, the sinews and tendons and the *dai mai* appear to share this function of providing dynamic tension for optimal growth.[1] *Zulinqi* GB-41 is also the point where the *qi* exits the Gall Bladder channel to connect with the Liver channel, which may be a further indication of the influence of the *dai mai* on horizontal integration as it shares this connection between two internally–externally related meridians.

Another correlation is seen in the flavor associated with the Wood element: sour. The main property associated with the sour flavor is that it astringes, which is also one of the main functions of the *dai mai*. Astringency plays a significant role in horizontal integration—the degree to which one is able to connect to the rest of humanity is dependent upon a strong vertical connection within oneself, which derives in part from the ability to contract and create boundaries. It is also this energy of contracting/astringing which pulls that which is experienced at the level of humanity into the interior to be integrated at the deepest level.

Further, there is a strong correlation between the *dai mai* and the *shaoyang*. Not only is the confluent point of

---

1   Proper nourishment is also vital. If there is Liver Blood deficiency, often the tendons and sinews become tense, and vice versa—if there is too much tension, it can block the proper flow of blood and lead to malnourishment (and therefore greater tension).

the *dai mai* located on the Gall Bladder Channel of Foot Shaoyang, but it is coupled with a point on the San Jiao Channel of Hand Shaoyang (*waiguan* SJ-5) in the master–couple system of opening the extraordinary meridians. Another correlation is seen in the way in which the *dai mai* divides and connects above and below and the inside and the outside, while the *shaoyang* level is said to be half interior, half exterior. The San Jiao also shares the function of linking the inside and the outside, and the *ying* and *wei*, and thus works intimately with the *dai mai* to balance horizontal integration.

The Three *Dantian* and Windows of Heaven, Earth, and Human

If the *dai mai* has the function of binding the meridians and providing dynamic structural flexibility, and through these functions affects the free flow of qi through the body, we can find this functional aspect of the *dai mai* present at various places throughout the body. In looking at the character "*dai*" (帶), it is shown as a piece of cloth (a hanging handkerchief or towel) below the pictograph of a belt with three pendants hanging from it. As discussed previously, the number three is often used to symbolize the trinity of Heaven, Earth, and Humanity as well as the three *dantian* and the three treasures of *jing*, *qi*, and *shen*. The "cloth" (巾) radical in the *dai* character may have significance as well: in anchoring all of the vertically flowing energy at this level and allowing each individual to be incarnated in a body, the *dai mai* may assist in providing the "cloth" or covering of a body for the spirit while it is here on Earth.

In looking at the character from this perspective, it seems plausible that the *dai mai* may be present not only at the level of the lower *dantian*, but may be energetically present at the level of the middle and upper *dantian* as well. This also makes sense in that, from one perspective, the three *dantian* are reflections of each other. This is supported in that *zulinqi* GB-41 is indicated for symptoms such as abdominal cramping, breast distension and tenderness, and headache, all of which correlate to the levels of the three *dantian*. Also, in the *Ode of the Obstructed River* are discussed the "Eight Therapeutic Methods" of using the confluent points of the extraordinary meridians to treat specific areas and symptoms. Here *zulinqi* GB-41 is indicated for disorders of the eyes, which may offer confirmation of the influence of the *dai mai* at the level of the upper dantian (as cited in Deadman and Al-Khafaji 2005).

Therefore, each *dantian* may be an energetic meeting point of the vertically flowing energy encircled by another energetic, circular pathway in the horizontal plane, which allows for spherical integrity at these major energy centers. If dynamic structural flexibility is the energetic aspect of being that allows one to expand and contract in relation to others and one's environment (and thus defines the boundaries of one's energy field and each *dantian*), spherical integration is the aspect that brings integration even as the boundaries are continuously shifting from moment to moment. These two aspects allow for a homeodynamic state of balance within each being.

Another way that the *dai mai* seems to be reflected throughout the body is at the three (or five) "windows"— the Windows of Heaven, Earth, and Humanity. The neck is well known as the Window of Heaven, as it is the connection between the head (Heaven) and the body, thus connecting the Macrocosmic Heaven (as reflected by the upper *dantian*) with the human body. The neck is a major place in the body where the meridians are "bottlenecked"—bound tightly together just as the *dai mai* binds the meridians. Similarly, one could say that there are Windows of Earth and Humanity, which would correspond to the hips and shoulders (or perhaps even the entirety of the legs and arms), respectively.[2] These are the connection between the Macrocosmic Earth *qi* and the lower *dantian* and the connection between the middle *dantian* and the rest of humanity.

Why are there two Windows of Earth and two Windows of Humanity, yet only one Window of Heaven? For Earth and Humanity exist in duality, while in Heaven there is unity. Thus we have two legs that correspond to the duality present at the level of Earth, two arms that correspond to the duality present at level of humanity, and only one head—which corresponds to the unity of Heaven. And, just as the *dai mai* binds all of the meridians flowing vertically within the body, at each of these "windows" all of the meridians are similarly constricted and bound.

This can be extended to include all of the joints, as the meridians are constricted and bound at every joint as they pass through. And, after all, what is the waist (the primary

---

2   Interestingly, one of the English definitions of "girdle" (as in Girdling Vessel) is the anatomical reference to the parts of the body that unite the upper or lower extremities with the axial skeleton—the shoulder and pelvic girdles. It should also be noted that Jeffrey Yuen refers to this connection between the Earth and the lower *dantian* as the "Doorways to the Earth," and discusses the relation of the Window of the Sky and Doorways to the Earth to the upper and lower sensory orifices (Yuen 2006).

location of the *dai mai*) but the largest "joint" in the body? If we look at the early Chinese anatomical positions (arms stretching up towards Heaven), then the joints line up in a way that allows a horizontal circle to flow around them. Although *zulinqi* GB-41 is not specifically indicated for pain or problems of the joints, it is interesting to note that *waiguan* SJ-5, the confluent point of the *yang wei mai* and the couple point of the *dai mai*, is a significant and often-used point for swelling, pain, and stiffness of the joints, shoulders, and neck (Deadman and Al-Khafaji 2005).

The *Zang*

The *dai mai* can also be seen as assisting with the dynamic structural flexibility necessary for the flourishing of the *zang*, or *yin* organs. The *zang* have the function of storing various vital substances/essences; therefore, they must be firm and strong, yet flexible enough to hold and release the vital substances as necessary. This "holding" is often thought of as a function of the Spleen—the Spleen is responsible for holding the blood in the vessels and the organs in their places. However, it is possible that there is a confluence of the *dai mai* and Spleen energies that carry out this function together. As stated by Larre and Rochat de la Vallée, "The ability of *dai mai* to hold and suspend is also very close to one of the functions of the spleen" (1997, p. 142). Thus, the *dai mai*'s function of dynamic structural flexibility may help to provide the structure for each individual organ. From one perspective, each of the organs (and especially the Heart) is a microcosmic reflection of the human, and therefore it makes sense that the structure of the individual organ would be provided by the *dai mai*, just as it provides the dynamic structural flexibility for the individual human being.

Just as we have seen a close association between the Liver and the *dai mai*, we can also see that there appears to be a strong link with the Spleen as well. Besides sharing the function of holding and suspending, we can also look at the point *zhangmen* LIV-13, which is the Front-*mu* of the Spleen, the *hui*-Meeting of the *zang*, and, according to some sources, the starting point of the *dai mai* (see the Appendix for the pathway of the *dai mai*). This implies that there is a coalescing of these three energies (Liver, Spleen, and *dai mai*) that, in turn, is responsible in part for the health and well-being of all of the *zang* organs. The connection between the *dai mai*, Spleen, and Liver is also supported by the classification of a *dai mai* pulse as being when the pulse is largest in both *guan* positions— that is, the positions associated with Liver and Spleen (see Morris 2002b for further information on the extraordinary vessel pulses).

This link between the *dai mai*, Spleen, and Liver is significant, as it relates to the ability of the *dai mai* to balance vertical and horizontal integration. Among the *zang*, the Liver is a *zang* that is primarily related to vertical integration, while the Spleen is a *zang* that is primarily related to horizontal integration—taking in and digesting that which we experience at the human/horizontal level of reality. In looking at the pulses, we also see these correspondences. As noted in Chapter 2, the pulse on the left wrist reflects the process of vertical integration, and the left middle position corresponds to the Liver and Gall Bladder, while the pulse on the right wrist corresponds to horizontal integration, and the right middle position corresponds to the Spleen and Stomach. Thus the Liver and Spleen can be seen as a central connection within the vertical and horizontal axes, respectively. The *dai mai*, in providing the balance between vertical and horizontal integration, is an integral part of balancing the Liver and Spleen energies. If the vertical connection is strong and clear (with the Liver *qi* flowing smoothly), and the horizontal connection is strong and clear (with the Spleen *qi* harmonious), it becomes easier to take in and process at the horizontal level and to let go of what is not needed.

Returning to the Source

One more aspect of the *dai mai* that is worth examining is its ability to guide the *qi* back to the Source. In the cycle of the evolution of consciousness, the one breaks into two, the two into three, and the three into the ten thousand things, before returning to a state of oneness. If the lower *dantian* relates to the source of the extraordinary vessels and the beginning of life, and it is to this source that we must return, then it appears that the *dai mai* has an integral role in bringing us back to this quiescent state.

The *dai mai* travels around the waist and binds the *ren*, *du*, and *chong mai* at the level of the lower *dantian*. As stated by Larre and Rochat de la Vallée:

> [The *dai mai*] also has a close relationship with the common origin of *du mai*, *ren mai* and *chong mai* which is in the *bao zhong* (胞中) or intimate envelope. Many commentators stress the influence of *dai mai* in making a complete connection with the first four extraordinary meridians in this area of the origin. (1997, p. 144)

These three meridians (*ren, du,* and *chong mai*) have been said to be the source of the other extraordinary meridians, as well as the source of the *zangfu* and primary channels. According to Li Shi Zhen, "The extraordinary vessels are the root of the Great Avenue of Pre-Heaven, the Governing, Directing and Penetrating Vessels [Du-Ren-Chong Mai] are the Source of Creation" (as cited in Maciocia 2005, p. 821). Yet the *dai mai* is not only connected to these meridians; it binds them and renders them whole again. The "*Dai Mai* is often referred to as the Meridian that maintains the integrity of the First Ancestries, that returns the integrity: the *Chong* in the middle, the *Ren* in the front, and the *Du* in the back" (Yuen 2005, p. 46).

If the *dai mai* relates to vertical and horizontal integration, it is likely that it plays a pivotal role in connecting post-heaven and pre-heaven. We saw above the strong correlation between the *dai mai* and Spleen (the source of post-heaven essence), as well as the importance of the astringing function of the *dai mai* in integrating at the deepest level that which is experienced at the level of humanity (transforming and transporting post-heaven to pre-heaven), and here we have a link between the *dai mai* and the extraordinary vessels at the lower *dantian* (the original pre-heaven). Therefore, it may be that the *dai mai* plays a role in connecting the post-heaven *qi* and essence of the Spleen with the pre-heaven *qi* and essence of the Kidneys at the Source. As stated by Larre and Rochat de la Vallée, the *dai mai* "conducts the *qi* of the whole organism in the correct direction and to its final destination" (1997, p. 148). Further support of this is found in that some have postulated that the *dai mai* connects to *shenshu* BL-23 (back-*shu* point of the Kidneys) and *mingmen* DU-4, points corresponding directly to the Kidneys and the lower *dantian*.

Conclusion

In this chapter we have explored some of the correspondences of the *dai mai* with the *zangfu* and primary channels. The *dai mai* seems to correspond to the circle of the *zhong* (中) character, the circular energy that is present throughout the universe and provides dynamic structural flexibility while allowing for spherical integration. The perfection of the circle and sphere is that all sides, every point, has dynamic tension, with equal energetic pressure both within and without. The *dai mai* is the energetic border (circular/spherical in nature) that keeps the dynamic tension and regulates expansion/contraction, pushing/pulling, and astringing/slackening of the individual in relation to their environment. The *dai mai* also guides the *qi* back to the Source, to the three extraordinary vessels that are the source of creation (*ren*, *du*, and *chong mai*).

Dynamic structural flexibility allows each individual to balance vertical and horizontal integration, connecting above and below and the inside and the outside in cycles of continuous growth and expansion. Trees, compared with other plants, are more firmly rooted and have a stronger vertical connection that enables them to be a greater channel for connecting Heaven and Earth. This strength enables them to stay true to themselves and to be of greater benefit to everything else around them. The *dai mai*, in providing this same circular/spherical integrity in human beings, assists one in staying true to oneself while connecting to everything else present at the level of humanity.

It is the interaction of Heaven and Earth that gives rise to the ten thousand things present at the level of humanity; every entity at this level is a coming together of these two polar energies, and thus it may be that everything in existence at the level of humanity is dependent upon a form of dynamic structural flexibility to exist at this level of reality. This spherical integrity of dynamic structural flexibility, which is present in every energetic field, allows each individual to be dynamically balanced in relation to their environment. For it is only through vertical integration that one gains the strength to expand horizontally, and it is only by integrating the inside and the outside that such strength has relevance. In this way, each individual can exist in a state of experiential awareness, staying true to self while experiencing the beautiful perfection of humanity. With the foundation of these first three chapters, we can now move on to examine possible relationships of the extraordinary vessels and the primary channels to aspects of Daoist cosmology and the evolution of consciousness.

Chapter 4

THE *YING QI* CYCLE AND A RELATION OF THE EXTRAORDINARY VESSELS TO DAOIST COSMOLOGY

The *ying qi* flows through the 12 primary channels, corresponding to the horary clock and the cycles of day and night. As it flows through the channels, it is following the cycle of birth, transformation, and death, just as the sun is born each morning and dies each night. If we follow the journey of the *ying qi* through the 12 primary channels, we find that it follows a course that moves from interior to exterior and exterior to interior, as well as connecting above and below. In so doing, it helps to maintain individual integrity while allowing one to connect Heaven and Earth, and the inside and the outside. This is the process of vertical and horizontal integration, the integration and connection of body and spirit, and self and other, which allows for nourishment, growth, and transformation in the day-to-day aspects of living. The *ying qi* cycle therefore corresponds closely to the process of the dynamic flow of *qi* at the level of humanity and the evolution of consciousness—expansion outward from the Source and the return to Source on a daily basis.

Compared with the primary channels, the extraordinary vessels correspond relatively more to macro-cycles and trends, to the constitutional aspects of being and our connection to pre-heaven. This is seen in the way in which the primary channels circulate *ying qi* while the extraordinary vessels have a closer association to *yuan qi* and *jing*. It is also of note that many Daoist practices have historically used the extraordinary vessels as a focus for spiritual practice and transformation (Deng 1990). Within the three primary forms of *qi* (*jing qi*, *ying qi*, and *wei qi*), *ying qi* corresponds to the middle level or pivot, and thus corresponds to the level of humanity.

While the extraordinary vessel confluent points are well known in acupuncture theory and practice, the significance and meaning of their placement along the primary channel system is rarely discussed; similarly, the interaction and direct connections between the primary channels and extraordinary vessels are generally viewed as fairly limited. However, given that very few acupuncture point category placements are arbitrary, it seems likely that the placement of the extraordinary vessel confluent points has a deeper meaning, and may even shed light on other connections between the extraordinary vessels and the primary channels.

In this chapter, we will follow the daily cycle of the *ying qi* through the primary channels, in order to examine the order in which the extraordinary vessels are theoretically accessed on a daily basis (according to when the *ying qi* passes their corresponding confluent points). In so doing, a relationship and pattern emerges that suggests an underlying coherency and structure in the nature of the extraordinary vessels themselves, as well as in their relation to the primary channels, concepts of Daoist cosmology, and the evolution of consciousness.

The Quiescent State

We begin our journey through the primary channels with the Lung Channel of Hand Taiyin. This meridian begins the cycle of *ying qi* through the 12 primary channels and corresponds to 3–5am, the pre-dawn of a new day. Starting in the middle *jiao* and emerging at *zhongfu* LU-1, the *ying qi* flows through the Lung channel and in its course passes through *lieque* LU-7, the confluent point of the *ren mai*. Thus the first extraordinary vessel that is theoretically accessed, at the "birth" of each new day, is the *ren mai*— that is, the "conception" vessel. Seen from this perspective, it is interesting to note Yang's commentary on the 28th Difficult Issue and the meaning of the character for *ren*: "*Jen* 任 ('controller') stands for *jen* 妊 ('pregnancy'). This is the basis of man's [coming to] life and nourishment" (Unschuld 1986, p. 329). Examined in light of the *ying qi* cycle and the placement of the confluent point of the *ren mai* in relation to this cycle, perhaps the *ren mai* also has a relation to each individual's "coming to life" each morning, as this is a microcosmic reflection of birth on a daily basis.

Continuing, the *ying qi* moves into the exterior-paired Large Intestine Channel of Hand Yangming, traveling from the hands to the face, and corresponding to 5–7am. Here it connects to the Stomach Channel of Foot Yangming, corresponding to 7–9am, where it flows all the way down to the feet and crosses over into the Spleen Channel of Foot Taiyin, corresponding to 9–11am. As the *ying qi* starts flowing up the Spleen channel, it passes *gongsun* SP-4, confluent point of the *chong mai*. In this first circuit of the horary cycle (corresponding to the first eight hours of the day, from 3am to 11am), the *ying qi* moves through the *taiyin* and *yangming* channels. It travels from the interior (Lung) to the exterior (Large Intestine–Stomach) and back to the interior (Spleen), and passes the confluent points that correspond to the *ren mai* and *chong mai*. This circuit and these four primary channels also define the *yin* (anterior) plane of the body; similarly, the *ren mai* and *chong mai* are also considered to be fundamentally *yin* meridians, given their close connections to the Uterus and the Sea of Blood, as well as their anatomical pathways.[1]

From the Spleen channel, the *ying qi* flows into the Heart Channel of Hand Shaoyin, corresponding to 11am–1pm, and marking the movement from the anterior plane of the body to the *yang* (posterior) plane of the body. After moving through the Heat channel, the *ying qi* flows into the Small Intestine Channel of Hand Taiyang, corresponding to 1–3pm. Here the *ying qi* passes the confluent point of the *du mai*, *houxi* SI-3. Flowing through the Small Intestine channel and passing the confluent point of the *du mai* also marks the completion of the first half of the horary cycle (the first

---

1   While the *chong mai* may be considered a *yin* meridian among the extraordinary vessels, it also has a fundamental relationship to the polarity between *yin* and *yang*, as will be seen shortly. However, in the context of pairing the extraordinary vessels (i.e. *ren/du*, *yin/yang qiao*, *yin/yang wei*, and *chong/dai*), the *chong mai* is the relatively *yin* vessel while the *dai mai* is the relatively *yang*.

six primary channels, Lung–Small Intestine, corresponding to 3am to 3pm), and corresponds to the *ying qi* passing the confluent points of the first three extraordinary vessels.

At this point in our journey we have passed the confluent points for, and theoretically accessed, the *ren*, *chong*, and *du mai*; these three vessels all start in the lower *dantian*, and can be considered three branches of one vessel (see Table 4.1; also see the Appendix for the pathways of these three vessels). According to Yü Shu's commentary (written in 1067) on the 28th Difficult Issue:

> Principally, the supervisor vessel {*du mai*}, the controller vessel {*ren mai*}, and the through-way vessel {*chong mai*} all three emerge from the *hui-yin* 會陰 hole, where they are united. One vessel, then, branches out into three [vessels], which proceed separately through the yin and yang sections [of the organism]. Hence, they all have different names. (Unschuld 1986, p. 330)

This concept of one vessel splitting into the three branches of the *ren*, *du*, and *chong mai* is significant, and points to a relationship between these three vessels and the original oneness as it divides into three.

Table 4.1 Confluent Points of the First Half of the Ying Qi *Cycle*

Ying qi cycle	Confluent points	Extraordinary vessel
LU–LI	*Lieque* LU-7	*Ren mai*
SP–ST	*Gonsun* SP-4	*Chong mai*
HE–SI	*Houxi* SI-3	*Du mai*

The trinity of the *ren–chong–du mai*, while still in a state of undifferentiated oneness in the lower *dantian*, can be referred to as the quiescent state—the deep interior reservoir from which all life springs forth. Thus they have a correspondence to the undifferentiated oneness as it is just beginning to separate into the foundations of *yin, yang*, and the pivot between; it is from this triad that all else comes into being—both in the macrocosmic universe as well as in the microcosm of the human body.

Therefore, the *ren mai* and *du mai* correspond to the deep polarity of *yin* and *yang* within the channel system, with the *chong mai* being the connection/pivot between them. In the macrocosmic trinity, the pivot corresponds to the level of humanity, within the *ren–chong–du mai* this would correspond to the *chong mai*. Within these three extraordinary vessels, the *ren mai* is often referred to as the Sea of Yin, while the *du mai* is often referred to as the Sea of Yang; thus the *chong mai* can be seen as the pivot between the *yin* and yang of the *ren* and *du mai*. It may be for this reason that the *chong mai* is called the Sea of Blood, the Sea of the 12 Channels, and the Sea of the *Zangfu*.

As noted by Kiiko Matsumoto and Stephen Birch, Li Shi Zhen stated that: "The ren mai and du mai make contact together at the chong mai." They go on to say that:

> He explains this statement by noting that the ren mai and du mai are the fundamental divisions of yin and yang in the body. The chong mai insures the inseparability of oneness of the ren and du mai, the yin and yang functions. (1986, p. 16)[2]

---

2   This concept is also expounded upon by Lonny Jarrett: "Note that chongmai (衝脈), one of the eight extra meridians, possesses the

Just as Humanity is found between Heaven and Earth, likewise the *chong mai* is found between the *ren* and *du mai*. Further support of this was seen in previous chapters, in that certain Daoist perspectives discuss a branch of the *chong mai* (sometimes referred to as the pre-heaven *chong mai*, the *zhong mai*, or the *taiji* pole) that runs straight through the center of the body, from *huiyin* REN-1 to *baihui* DU-20, connecting the three *dantian* and anterior (*ren*) and posterior (*du*) heaven (see Yuen 2005 and Deng 1990).

The relationship of the *chong mai* to connecting pre-heaven and post-heaven is significant, in that it shows a further relationship of this extraordinary vessel to being the pivot or meeting point between polarities. As stated by Maciocia, in describing the *chong mai*:

> It is described as the Sea of the five Yin and six Yang organs as it is a fundamental vessel that connects the Pre-Heaven and the Post-Heaven Qi, owing to its connection with Kidneys and Stomach. It is connected to the Kidneys as it originates in that area and it distributes Essence all over the body. It is connected to the Stomach as it passes through the point ST-30 Qichong, which is a point for the Sea of Food. (2005, pp. 850–851)

---

function of blending the influences of heaven and earth, and yin and yang, as they are mediated by the conception and governor vessels, respectively" (2004, p. 8).

Further, as Larre and Rochat de la Vallée write:

> When you take *chong mai* it appears to be both the link
> between and the manifestation of a couple, *yin* and
> *yang*, blood and *qi*, etc. and also the connection between
> posterior and anterior heaven, stomach and kidneys. It
> is also able to unify the three levels of the body, the
> three heaters. (1997, p. 121)

This relationship of the *chong mai* to pre-heaven and post-heaven may shed light on the name of *gongsun* SP-4, the confluent point of the *chong mai*. *Gongsun* is often translated as "Grandfather Grandson;" if the *chong mai* is a primary link between pre-heaven and post-heaven, and therefore between the Kidneys and Spleen, then perhaps *gongsun* refers to this very relationship between the Kidneys and Spleen. In the five-phase relationship between these *zangfu*, the Spleen is the "Grandfather" of the Kidneys.

It is from this quiescent state of the *ren–chong–du mai*, the original division of the oneness into the three of *yin*, yang and the connection/pivot between these two polar aspects, that everything else comes into existence.[3] This concept of the *ren–chong–du mai* as the *taiji* or "supreme polarity" is graphically illustrated below in Figure 4.1.

---

3   Also see Su Wen (Simple Questions) chapter 60: "Among the eight extraordinary channels, the ren/conception, du/governing and chong/vitality are of the greatest importance" (Ni 1995, p. 209).

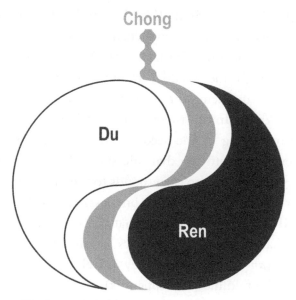

Figure 4.1 The Quiescent State

This perspective on the relationship between the *ren, chong,* and *du mai* may also provide further illumination on the name given to this extraordinary vessel, the *chong mai,* that mediates between *du* and *ren mai,* Heaven and Earth, pre-heaven and post-heaven, and *yin* and *yang. Chong* is often translated as "penetrating;" perhaps it is given this name as it is this vessel which allows the interpenetration of these various polar aspects of *yin* and *yang* present throughout the body.

The Second Half of the Horary Cycle: Movement, Manifestation, and Integration

As we return to following the *ying qi* through its horary cycle, it enters the Bladder Channel of Foot Taiyang, corresponding to 3–5pm. This also marks the movement into the second six primary channels, corresponding to the time period from 3pm to 3am. As the *ying qi* flows down through the Bladder channel, it passes *shenmai* BL-62, the confluent point of the *yang qiao mai*, the Yang Motility Vessel. In this theoretical model, this corresponds to the beginning of the second order, moving from the quiescent state into the dynamic state of movement and manifestation. This also corresponds to the movement from the vertical axis (and relative oneness) to the horizontal axis and duality—thus we see that the next extraordinary vessels have more characteristics of duality (they have *yin* and *yang* components, they travel bilaterally rather than on the midline (see Appendix), and so forth). In the master–couple system, *shenmai* BL-62 is coupled with *houxi* SI-3, confluent point of the *du mai*. This suggests that the movement and mobilization of *yang*, the dynamic *yang*, arises out of the quiescent *yang*. Therefore, the *yang qiao mai*, the Yang Motility Vessel, may be seen as arising from the *du mai*, the Sea of Yang. As stated by Larre and Rochat de la Vallée, "the *qiao mai* follow the same pattern as the *du mai* and *ren mai*… They are just a development of the *du mai* and *ren mai*" (1997, p. 204). In a sense, the *du mai* can be seen as the *yin* within *yang* of these two coupled channels, pertaining to the deep, interior, quiescent state of *yang*, with the *yang qiao mai* representing the *yang* within *yang*, pertaining to the relatively more dynamic, active state of *yang* within the body.

Soon after passing *Shenmai* BL-62, the *ying qi* passes into the Kidney Channel of Foot Shaoyin, corresponding to 5–7pm. As it begins flowing up the Kidney channel, it

passes *zhaohai* K-6, confluent point of the *yin qiao mai*—
the Yin Motility Vessel. *Zhaohai* K-6 is paired with *lieque*
LU-7, confluent point of the *ren mai*—thus the movement
and mobilization of *yin*, the dynamic *yin*, may be seen as
arising out of the quiescent *yin*. Here again, the *ren mai*
would pertain to the *yin* within *yin* of these two coupled
channels (pertaining to the deep, interior, quiescent state
of *yin*, the Sea of Yin), and the *yin qiao mai* to the *yang*
within *yin* (pertaining to the relatively more dynamic,
active state of *yin*).

This close relationship between the *du mai* and the *yang
qiao mai*, and the *ren mai* and the *yin qiao mai*, is also reflected
in the way in which they were sometimes interchanged in
the classics. For examples of this, see the commentaries on
the 26th Difficult Issue, where they discuss which of the
extraordinary vessels have network vessels—in the *Nei Jing*
(Inner Classic) it is stated that it is the *ren* and the *du mai*
that have network vessels, whereas in the *Nan Jing* (Classic
of Difficult Issues) it is the *qiao mai*. In trying to clarify this,
Liao P'ing states: "Yang walker vessel must refer here to the
supervisor [vessel]. *The names are identical but the substance
is different.* [Yin walker vessel] must refer to the controller
[vessel]" (Unschuld 1986, p. 320; emphasis added).

After beginning in the lower dantian with the *ren*,
chong, and *du mai*, this movement of the *ying qi* through
the Bladder and Kidney channels would thus correspond
to the mobilization of the fundamental *yin* and *yang* of the
body through the activation of the *yin* and *yang qiao mai*.
This is also seen in basic Chinese physiology—in order for
the essence and *yuan qi* of the Kidneys and lower *dantian* to
nourish and sustain the function and structure of the human

being, it must first transform into *yin* and *yang*, which, once mobilized, go out to become the basis of the *yin* and *yang* for the *zangfu* and the entire body. In the daily evolutionary cycle of the extraordinary vessels, this mobilization of *yin* and *yang* may correspond to the opening of the *qiao mai*.

The relation of the *qiao mai* to this transformation may also be inferred from the literature:

> The commentators of the Nan jing and other texts suggest that the *zang* and the innermost are irrigated by the *yin qiao mai*, and the *fu* are watered by the *yang qiao mai*. This is just another way to show the total impregnation in the rising up movement of the *yin* and *yang* of the body. This could be interpreted as the *zang* and the *fu*, or the inner and outer parts of the body, or the front and the back—all interpretations are possible, because the main function of the *qiao mai* is to rule the exchanges and to create equilibrium between the *yin* and the *yang* at every level. (Larre and Rochat de la Vallée 1997, p. 174)

And as stated by Chang Shih-hsien, in commentating on the 26th Difficult Issue, "The yang walker [vessel] penetrates the five palaces; it masters the external [affairs]. The yin walker [vessel] links and penetrates the five depots; it masters the internal [affairs]" (Unschuld 1986, p. 319). We therefore see a close association between the actions of the *yin* and *yang qiao mai* and the mobilization of the essence from the lower *dantian* to generate and nourish the *zangfu* organs and the rest of the body.

At this point in the daily cycle, *yin* and *yang* may be moving, circulating, and manifesting throughout the body, creating the energetic polarity of body and spirit (and *jing* and *shen*) as it dynamically moves, weaves, and manifests throughout the body. In terms of Daoist cosmogenesis, this relates to the interpenetration of *yin* and *yang* as each individuated being becomes a conduit for the exchange of *yang qi* from Heaven and *yin qi* from Earth—it is the movement and interplay of *yin* and *yang* that occurs once the vertical foundation of division into three (Heaven–Humanity–Earth, or *ren–chong–du mai*) is established.

The movement of the *ying qi* through the Kidney channel marks the end of the second circuit of the horary clock (corresponding to the second eight hours of the day, from 11am to 7pm), during which time the *ying qi* moves through the *shaoyin* and *taiyang* meridians. This circuit and these four primary channels define the *yang* (posterior) plane of the body; during this part of the journey the *ying qi* passes the confluent points that correspond to the *du mai* and the two aspects of the *qiao mai*. The *du mai* is fundamentally *yang* in nature; similarly, the *qiao mai* (as a whole) may be considered to be fundamentally *yang*, given their close connections to the movement and mobilization of the quiescent *yin* and *yang*, not to mention their direct relationship to allowing each individual the ability to be active and physically move through the world.

Continuing along the horary cycle, the *ying qi* flows from the Kidney channel into the Pericardium Channel of Hand Jueyin, corresponding to 7–9pm. As the *ying qi* flows through the Pericardium channel, it passes *neiguan* P-6, which is the confluent point of the *yin wei mai*, the Yin/ Interior Linking vessel. In master–couple theory, *neiguan* P-6 is coupled with *gongsun* SP-4, the confluent point of the *chong mai*. Just as we saw above that the *yang qiao mai* and *yin qiao mai* may arise from the quiescent *yang* and *yin* of the *du* and *ren mai*, respectively, as seen through the coupling of their confluent points, so too does the *yin wei mai* appear to share a similar relationship to the *chong mai*. Just as the *chong mai* is the energetic polarity or pivot of the quiescent *yin* and *yang* of the *ren* and *du mai*, the *yin wei mai* may play a role as the energetic polarity of the mobilized *yin* and *yang* of the *yin* and *yang qiao mai*. The Yin Linking Vessel may thus allow the dynamic polarity of the *yin* and *yang qiao mai* to be integrated, thereby rendering the interior an integrated whole. Support for this is also seen in the pathology associated with the *yin wei mai*, as seen in the *Nan Jing* (Classic of Difficult Issues): "When the yin tie has an illness, one suffers from heartache" (Unschuld 1986, p. 333). The Heart symbolizes the one of the deepest unities of *yin* and *yang* within the human being, and corresponds to the middle *dantian*; heartache (whether physical or emotional) is often associated with a separation of *yin* and *yang*, a loss of integrity within self.

After each of the ten thousand things is made manifest through the interaction of the mobilized *yin* and *yang*, each individuated entity must integrate these polar energies to become whole within oneself before extending to connect with all else that is manifest; this can be seen as the action of the *yin wei mai* and the Heart. It may be at this point of the evolutionary cycle that one is able to experience self-realization as the *yin wei mai* engenders integration within oneself (see Figure 4.2).

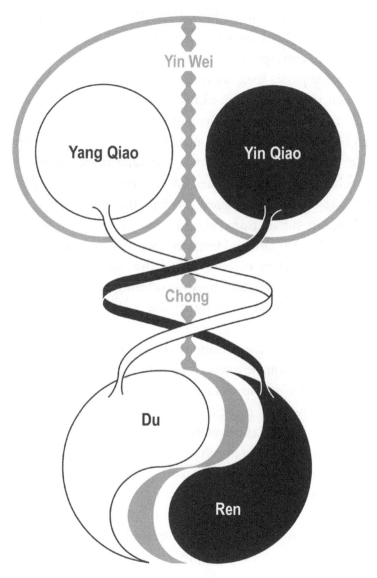

Figure 4.2 Manifestation and Self-Realization

After finishing its flow through the Pericardium channel, the *ying qi* flows into the San Jiao Channel of Hand Shaoyang, corresponding to 9–11pm. As it moves up the channel, it passes *waiguan* SJ-5, confluent point of the *yang wei mai*, the Yang/Exterior Linking vessel. The *yang wei mai* rules the exterior and movement towards the exterior, and can be seen as the energetic matrix of one's external energy field.[4] This is also supported when looking at the pathology associated with the *yang wei mai*, as seen in the *Nan Jing* (Classic of Difficult Issues): "When the yang tie has an illness, one suffers from [fits of] cold and heat" (Unschuld 1986, p. 333). Chills and fever are seen primarily in exterior pathologies, when the *wei qi* and the outermost level of the body is being affected—thus offering confirmation of a relationship between the *yang wei mai* and the external energetic field.

If the *yang wei mai* relates to the external level of being, and rules movement towards the exterior, then it will have a strong relationship to how each individual connects to others at the level of humanity. In the theories of Daoist cosmogenesis and the evolution of consciousness we have examined thus far, connecting to others (and all else that is present at the level of humanity) is the next step after each individuated being is integrated within themselves. It is only after the internal integration (as represented by the *yin wei mai* in this model) that one is able to then extend to connect to the exterior (as represented by the *yang wei mai*),

---

4   Also see Li Shi Zhen: "Hence, the *yang wei* governs the exterior of the entire body while the *yin wei* governs the interior of the entire body, and so they are referred to as *qian* and *kun*" (Chase and Shima 2010, p. 96).

thereby connecting the inside and the outside in a process of horizontal integration. As noted by Larre and Rochat de la Vallée, in referencing the work of Zhang Zicong, "This commentator also said that as the *qi* of *yin* and *yang qiao* are joined together, the exterior and interior are in an exchange and relationship and penetrate one another" (1997, p. 182). This may be read as suggesting that it is only after the joining/integration of the *qiao mai* (which, in this model, relates to the activation and function of the *yin wei mai*) that the *yang wei mai* opens to the exterior and the *wei mai* are able to connect with each other and allow interpenetration of the inside and the outside. Just as the *yin wei mai*, the "interior linking vessel," is the pivot between *yin* and *yang* within the individual human body (as relates to the integration of the *yin qiao mai* and *yang qiao mai*), the *yang wei mai*, or "exterior linking vessel," is the pivot between the *yin* and *yang* of the individual and the environment, between the inside and the outside.

The Return to Quiescence

Returning to the horary cycle, we near the end of our journey as the *ying qi* flows into and through the Gall Bladder Channel of Foot Shaoyang, corresponding to 11pm–1am. Traveling through this channel it passes *zulinqi* GB-41, confluent point of the *dai mai*, the Belt/Girdling Vessel. In this model, the activation of the *dai mai* may correspond to reaching a state of wholeness and completion, and of returning to the beginning to start the cycle anew. As seen in Chapter 3, one of the functions of the *dai mai* is to take one from the most expanded exterior state back to the deepest interior, back to the quiescent state. It is able to accomplish this through its actions of dynamic structural stability and spherical integration, thereby binding all of the meridians and the external energy field. In so doing, the *dai mai* is able to astringe the exterior and hold everything together in the horizontal plane, and from this place guide the *qi* back to the Source and the lower *dantian*. See Table 4.2 for the placement of each of the confluent points of the extraordinary vessels along the *ying qi* cycle.

Table 4.2 Confluent Points along the Ying Qi *Cycle*

Ying qi cycle	Confluent points	Extraordinary vessel
LU–LI	LU-7	Ren mai
SP–ST	SP-4	Chong mai
HE–SI	SI-3	Du mai
K–BL	BL-62, K-6	Qiao mai
P–SJ	P-6, SJ-5	Wei mai
LIV–GB	GB-41	Dai mai

If the *yang wei mai* is seen as the energetic matrix of the energy field that expands externally in relation to oneself in order to experience all that is present in one's environment, the *dai mai* may be seen as regulating how much horizontal expansion occurs. As stated by Larre and Rochat de la Vallée, "*Dai mai* is not only a circle but the expression of the volume of the body... The *dai mai* comes from within, and expands, giving an expansion of volume, and also a limit to this expansion" (1997, p. 154). The *dai mai* is also known to bind the *ren, chong,* and *du mai* (at the level of the lower *dantian*) and may thus act to bring each individuated being full circle: back to the beginning of undifferentiated oneness, back to the quiescent state. Further evidence of this is seen in Li Shi Zhen's work, the *Qi Jing Ba Mai Kao*: "Zhang Zi-He says that... The three vessels of the *chong*, *ren*, and *du* have the same origins but their trajectories differ. They are of a single source but have three branches and all network with the *dai* vessel" (Chase and Shima 2010, pp. 156–157). This is a return to the primordial unity that is reflected by the essence prior to division into *yin* and *yang*, a grounding back in the *yuan qi* and the Source.

Therefore, the *dai mai* may help to render the *yin* and *yang* aspects of being (above and below, inside and outside) into a unified whole and allow one to start the cycle again the next day. From this perspective it is interesting to note that, in Neoclassical Pulse Diagnosis, there is a dominant tendency for individuals to have a *dai mai* pulse (which occurs when the middle position on either wrist is the largest or most superficial) and/or a *yang wei mai* pulse (when there are ulnar displacements of the proximal positions with radial displacements of the distal positions) according to the eight extraordinary vessels system, as well as a tendency for a Liver-to-Lung blockage along the *ying qi* cycle.[5] These three pulse patterns correspond to the end of the *ying qi* cycle, when one is just on the verge of transitioning back to the interior and pre-heaven state. In modern society, the individual's energy is often "exteriorized" and drawn outward, and there is difficulty in guiding the *qi* back to the Source and returning to the quiescent state—thus it

---

5   For more information on this relationship, and extraordinary vessel pulse diagnosis, see Morris 2009.

makes sense that many individuals would have stagnations and challenges along these patterns.[6]

The *dai mai*, although theoretically activated at the end of the horary cycle, would therefore also relate to the beginning and to oneness. Within the extraordinary vessels there are four nuclear vessels (*ren, chong, du,* and *dai mai*) that relate primarily to the quiescent state, oneness, and the vertical axis, and they are paired (in the master–couple system) with four peripheral vessels (the *qiao* and *wei mai*) that primarily relate to the active/manifest state and expansion from the Source outwards, duality, and the horizontal axis. This perspective also lends itself to seeing how the *chong* and *dai mai* make a perfect *yin–yang* pair. The *chong mai* connects anterior and posterior heaven (*ren* and *du mai*), as it is the polarity between the two, whereas the *dai mai* wraps around the outside and contains them. Just as the *chong mai*, as the polarity between the *ren* and the *du mai*, becomes the link between the quiescent state and the dynamic state (and therefore corresponds to the movement from pre-heaven to post-heaven), so too does the *dai mai* relate to the movement from the dynamic state back to the quiescent state (corresponding to the movement from post-heaven back to pre-heaven).

---

6   Interestingly, this may also shed further light on the name of *zulinqi* GB-41—Foot Governor of Tears or Close to Tears. The end of a cycle, the death, the transition from the end of something to a new beginning is difficult, and often sad.

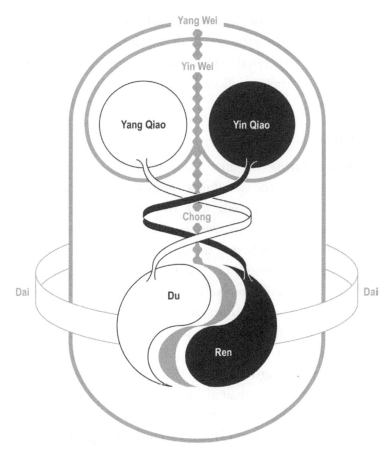

Figure 4.3 Connecting the Interior and Exterior, Returning to the Source

After passing through the Gall Bladder channel, the *ying qi* enters the Liver Channel of Foot Jueyin to finish its daily cycle, corresponding to 1–3am. This marks the movement through the third and final circuit of the *ying qi* cycle, corresponding to the meridians that define the pivotal (median/sagittal) plane of the body (*jueyin* and *shaoyang*). During this circuit the *ying qi* passes the confluent points corresponding to the *wei mai* and the *dai mai*; these meridians also have a strong resonance and association to being pivots/polarities by linking the inside and the outside and allowing the entire cycle of extraordinary vessels to become one integrated whole. See Figure 4.3 for a graphic illustration of these relationships.

Conclusion

To recap, during the first half of the horary cycle the *ying qi* passes the confluent points corresponding to the extraordinary vessels that have their origin in the lower *dantian*—the *ren*, *chong*, and *du mai*. These three extraordinary vessels are three yet one—they are three branches of one vessel, and are a reflection of the oneness as it divides into the triad of Heaven, Earth, and Humanity. Thereafter, the *ying qi* passes the confluent points of the *qiao mai*, which, in this model, correspond to the mobilization of the quiescent *yin* and *yang*, the dynamic *yin* and *yang* that moves through the body to nourish the *zangfu* and manifest each individuated being. Next, the cycle of the *ying qi* passes the confluent point of the *yin wei mai*, which assists in linking, consolidating, and integrating the internal manifestation of the dynamic *yin* and *yang* of the *qiao mai*. The internal integration of *yin* and *yang* then allows one to extend and connect within and without, as represented by the opening of the *yang wei mai*. Finally, the exterior can be consolidated and regulated as the *ying qi* cycles through the Gall Bladder channel and passes the confluent point of the *dai mai*, which also then facilitates the return to the quiescent state and oneness, allowing one to start the cycle again the next day.

This cycle of the extraordinary vessels corresponds to Daoist conceptions of cosmogenesis and the evolution of consciousness, and the processes of vertical and horizontal integration, and corresponds to the dynamic flow of *qi* at the level of humanity. Through this progression, one eventually returns to a state of oneness.

Chapter 5

PAIRING THE EXTRAORDINARY VESSELS AND THE EXTRAORDINARY ORGANS

In this chapter, I will continue building this model by examining a theoretical pairing of the extraordinary organs with the extraordinary vessels, similar to the way in which the *zangfu* are paired with the primary channels. It is my intent to put forward a perspective in which these seemingly disparate aspects of the medicine may be seen with a greater degree of integration, not only within themselves but also with the other foundational aspects of Chinese medicine. To explore this idea, I will look at correspondences between the extraordinary vessels and the extraordinary organs using the perspective of the three *dantian* and the three treasures, as well as structural, functional, and relational correspondences.

Correspondences between the Extraordinary Vessels and Organs

Although not much discourse about the relationship between the extraordinary vessels and the extraordinary organs can be found in the literature, there are several authors who discuss the correspondences in part. For example, both Maciocia (2005) and Jeffrey Yuen (2005) mention connections. These correspondences are, however, fairly general, and indicate several overlaps between the extraordinary vessels and the extraordinary organs. According to Yuen (2005), connections can be seen between the Brain and the *du*, *qiao*, and *ren mai*; between the Uterus and the *ren*, *chong*, *du*, and *dai mai*; and between the Gall Bladder and the *dai* and *wei mai*, among others. Maciocia (2005) also offers the following correspondences: Brain: *du* and *qiao mai*; Uterus: *chong* and *ren mai*; Blood vessels: *chong mai*; Gall Bladder: *dai mai*; Marrow: *chong* and *du mai*; Bones: *chong*, *du*, and *ren mai*.

Many of these connections come from the pathways of the vessels, as well as confluence of function. However, it is also possible that there is a one-to-one correspondence between the extraordinary vessels and organs, that they pertain to each other similarly to the way that the primary channels and *zangfu* pertain to each other. Nor is this in conflict with the correspondences put forth by Yuen, Maciocia, and others. It is quite possible that there are overlapping correspondences of several extraordinary vessels to a given extraordinary organ at the same time that there is a primary, one-to-one correspondence—just as there are sometimes several primary meridians that will pass through or relate to any given *zangfu*, at the same time that there are primary correspondences between each *zang* and *fu* and its related channel.

At first this may not seem plausible, as there are eight extraordinary channels, while only six extraordinary organs. However, in many of the classics the *yin* and *yang qiao mai* are simply referred to as the *qiao mai*, and similarly for the *wei mai*. Therefore, for purposes of this model, I will place the *yin* and *yang* aspects of the *qiao* and *wei mai* each together as one channel, similar to the way in which each interiorly–exteriorly related primary channel pair corresponds to one set of *zangfu*. This would then leave us with six extraordinary vessels, which makes it possible to pair the extraordinary vessels and the extraordinary organs together in a one-to-one correspondence. To examine these theoretical pairings, I will first examine the Uterus, Blood Vessels, and Brain together as a set, and then turn to the Marrow, Bones, and Gall Bladder.

The Three *Dantian*: Uterus, Blood Vessels, and Brain

The perspective of the three *dantian* provides a perfect lens through which to examine the correspondences of the Uterus, Brain, and Blood Vessels with three of the extraordinary vessels—the *ren mai*, *du mai*, and *chong mai*, respectively. As seen previously, within the three *dantian*, the lower *dantian* is in correspondence with Earth, the upper dantian is in correspondence with Heaven, and the middle *dantian* is in correspondence with Humanity; together these three *dantian* correspond to the vertical axis of integration.

This trinity is also reflected in the three treasures of *jing*, *qi*, and *shen*. *Jing* is the dense, material, *yin* substance, the essence, the physical basis for experiential reality that corresponds to Earth and the lower *dantian*. *Shen* is the ethereal, the spirit, the pure awareness that corresponds to Heaven, *yang*, and the upper *dantian*. *Qi* is the connection between *jing* and *shen* in the process of internal alchemy, and regulates the connection between above and below and the inside and the outside (vertical and horizontal integration) and thus corresponds to Humanity and the middle *dantian*—the pivot of the dynamic flow of *qi* at the level of humanity.

As the extraordinary organs relate to the deep, constitutional, pre-heaven aspects of being, it makes sense that they would have direct correspondences to the three *dantian* and the three treasures, which are foundational aspects in the formation and physiology of the human being. As noted by Larre and Rochat de la Vallée, the extraordinary organs "are closer to the original formation of the body, and they are also more ancient, primitive and deep and more able to ensure the continuity of life" (2003, p. 205). Looking at it from this perspective, it is of note that the literature (as well as the anatomy of the body) suggests that the Uterus corresponds to the lower *dantian* and *jing*, and the Brain corresponds to the upper *dantian* and *shen*. As noted by Yuen, "The *Jing* Essence begins in the level of the Uterus" (2006, p. 69).[1] And Li Shi Zhen stated that, "The Brain is the Palace of the Original Shen" (as cited in Maciocia 2005, p. 231).

---

1   It should be noted that the Uterus, as an extraordinary *fu*, is present in both men and women: "The Uterus was called *Zi Bao* in Chinese medicine. *Bao* is actually a structure that is common to both men and women and is in the Lower Field of Elixir (*Dan Tian*): in men, *Bao* is the 'Room of Essence;' in women, it is the Uterus" (Maciocia 2005, p. 225).

Which extraordinary organ would then be in correspondence with the middle *dantian*? Again, in looking at the literature as well as anatomical correspondences, it seems clear that the Blood Vessels are the extraordinary organ that corresponds directly to the middle *dantian*. It is at the level of the middle *dantian* that we find the Heart and the greatest concentration of *mai*—the blood vessels of cardio-pulmonary circulation as well as the major vessels relating to systemic circulation. Further, it has been said that "the Blood Vessels are primarily influenced by the Heart as this governs Blood and controls blood vessels, but also by the Lungs as they control all channels and vessels" (Maciocia 2005, p. 233), and also that, "There is a strong relationship between the mai and the heart because the heart is the master of the mai" (Larre and Rochat de la Vallée 2003, p. 108), both of which point to the middle *dantian* as the center of the Blood Vessels. It is also from the Heart and the middle *dantian* that there are blood vessels regulating circulation between the Heart and the Brain (upper *dantian*) as well as between the Heart and the Uterus (lower *dantian*). Therefore, it is possible that the lower, middle and upper *dantian* (and *jing*, *qi* and *shen*) correspond to the Uterus, Blood Vessels, and Brain, respectively.

The Seas of *Jing*, *Qi*, and *Shen: Ren*, *Chong*, and *Du Mai*

As seen previously, the *ren* and *du mai* may be seen as the fundamental division of *yin* and *yang* within the channel system, corresponding to the deep, interior Source as it is just beginning to form the polarity of Earth and Heaven within the human being. If we look at the *ren* and *du mai* in relation to the three treasures and the three *dantian*, we can see that the *ren mai*, in being the Sea of *Yin*, has a strong correspondence to Earth, *jing*, the lower *dantian*, and the Uterus. Similarly, we can see that the *du mai*, in being the Sea of *Yang*, has a strong correspondence to Heaven, *shen*, the upper *dantian*, and the Brain. These associations are reinforced by the *ren mai*'s direct connection to the Uterus, and the *du mai*'s direct connection to the Brain (see Appendix). In discussing *Nan Jing* Difficulty 28, Larre and Rochat de la Vallée state that:

> In this description the text says the *du mai*…enters the brain with a *shu* (屬) relationship. *Shu* represents the idea of belonging to something… In the description of each of the twelve meridians this relationship of belonging is the special connection between a meridian and its viscera, and the *luo* (络) relationship is the special relationship with the coupled viscera… The relationship of the *du mai* with the brain is both *luo* and *shu*… It is exactly as if the *du mai* is the link to the brain in all ways. (2003, pp. 39–40)

The lower and upper *dantian* are reflections of each other, just as the *ren* and *du mai* mirror each other; each pair forms a polarity of *yin* and *yang*, body/*jing* and spirit/*shen*. As noted by Yuen, "You see the mirror image between the Uterus and the Brain, between *Ren* and its connection to the *Du*, *Yin* and *Yang* giving birth to each other in many ways" (2006, p. 74).

For this reason, the *ren mai* could perhaps be called the Sea of *Jing*, and the *du mai* the Sea of *Shen*. This would then help in explaining why, in the history of Chinese medicine, some have said that the Brain is the residence of the *shen*, while others have said that the Heart is the residence of the *shen*. If instead we think of the *du mai* as the Sea of *Shen*, and understand that the *du mai* has an intimate connection with all three *dantian*, then it becomes clear that all three of these areas are major concentrations of awareness/*shen*, and that the *du mai* may assist in the movement of the *shen* between these major energetic centers.

The *du mai* is said to start in the lower *dantian*, has a channel that passes through the Heart and Kidneys (making it the only extraordinary vessel to pass through a *zangfu* organ), and directly connects to the Brain—the three areas that correspond directly to the levels of the three *dantian* (see Appendix). As stated by Maciocia, "Thus, the Governing Vessel has a strong influence on the mental-emotional state because it is the channel connection between the Kidneys, Heart and Brain" (2005, p. 843). Considering that the Blood houses the *shen*, it is also of note that the three *dantian* (Uterus, Heart/Blood Vessels, and Brain) are also major areas of blood circulation.

As seen above, with all polarities, there is something that simultaneously connects and separates the *yin* and *yang* aspects of the *ren* and *du mai*: the *chong mai*. In the model of the three *dantian*, the *chong mai* then takes its place in correspondence with the level of humanity—the middle *dantian*. This also corresponds to the level of *qi* in the three treasures, and the Blood Vessels in the extraordinary organs. From this perspective, it is interesting to note that the *chong mai* has variously been referred to as the Sea of Blood, the Sea of the Five *Zang* and the Six *Fu*, and the Sea of the 12 Channels, and is said to be able to treat blood stagnation anywhere in the body. As stated by Maciocia:

Apart from the gynaecological system, the Blood of the whole body relies for its movement and circulation on the Penetrating Vessel. Being the Sea of Blood and the Sea of the 12 Channels, the Penetrating vessel controls all the Blood Connecting channels. The Blood Connecting channels are the deep level of the Connecting (*Luo*) channels, a level that is connected with Blood and blood vessels...the Penetrating Vessel can be used to treat Blood stasis...anywhere in the body. (2005, p. 856)

Further, as written by Larre and Rochat de la Vallée, "The *chong mai* is implicated wherever there is something wrong with the circulation, not just involving one or two meridians, but more generally" (1997, p. 128). Thus, there is a very close and intimate relationship between the *chong mai*, the Blood Vessels, and blood circulation, and it is quite feasible that the *chong mai* and Blood Vessels have a direct relationship to each other.

It is also of note that one of the indications of *gongsun* SP-4 (confluent point of the *chong mai*) is heart pain, and also that one of the pathways of the *chong mai* disperses in the chest region (see Appendix). Therefore, we can see that there are significant and direct correspondences between the *ren*, *chong*, and *du mai* with the Uterus, Blood Vessels, and Brain, respectively; these pairings resonate with the three *dantian* and the three treasures, and thus correspond to the vertical axis of integration within the body.

Qiao Mai and Marrow: Global Nourishment by the Essence

"*Qiao*" is often translated as motility. If the "*yin*" and "*yang*" *qiao mai* are related to the motility and movement of *yin* and *yang*, they can be seen as having a strong relation to the mobilization of the essence as it arises from the Source, as seen in the previous chapter. In Chinese physiology, the essence first transforms into *yin* and *yang*, which then go out to become the basis of *yin* and *yang* throughout the entire body. Similarly, the Marrow is often discussed as a mobile form of the essence—the essence that fills the spinal cord, Brain, and bony cavities and "moves" through the body. As stated by Larre and Rochat de la Vallée:

> In books of the same period there is a definition of marrow as a great liquid which flows. One of the differences between the brain and the marrow is that the brain is like a sea, immobile and fixed…but what flows into the sea is circulating and this is the marrow, the *qi*, the nourishment, the meridians and the blood… One of the main functions of the marrow is to circulate and irrigate, to flow into the bones, the skull, the hollows and the orifices. This is the movement of the marrow inside the bones. (2003, pp. 92–93)

Thus both the *qiao mai* and the Marrow are closely related to the movement of essence through the body.

While the Brain as an extraordinary organ corresponds to the *du mai*, it may be that the *qiao mai* are responsible, in part, for nourishing the Brain. This is seen in the pathway of the *qiao mai*—both start at the malleoli, and from here flow up to meet at *jingming* BL-1 and enter the Brain (see Appendix):

> The *qiao mai* represent the first division and repartition of *yin* and yang…with a meeting point not only at the inner corner of the eyes but also in the depths of the brain. Beginning in the middle of the heel they touch the power of the earth. They provide a kind of rooting in the earth, and taking from below the forces to make all the earthly *qi*, the *yin*, essences, water and nutritive power rise up inside the body. (Larre and Rochat de la Vallée 1997, p. 203)

This is also reinforced by the name of this point:

> *Jing ming* (睛 明) gives the idea both of light and of the illumination coming from irrigation by the essences. *Jing*…is refering to nothing other than the gathering together of the essences (*jing* 精) of the five *zang* and the six *fu*… This is another way to show how all the vitality is brought to the upper orifices and to the brain by the workings of the *qiao mai*. (Larre and Rochat de la Vallée 1997, p. 173)

Therefore, the *qiao mai* may be seen as carrying the essence from "Earth" (which includes both the macrocosmic Earth and the lower *dantian*) up to the Brain, the Sea of Marrow. This process also reflects the movement of Marrow up to the Brain: "The commentators said that the marrow circulates following the hollows inside the bones, and thus rises up to be in free communication with the brain" (Larre and Rochat de la Vallée 2003, p. 97). Clearly, both the *qiao mai* and the Marrow may have an intimate relationship to global nourishment by the essence, and particularly the nourishment of the Brain.

It is also of note that the Marrow is sometimes referred to as *jing* plus *shen* (Yuen 2006), which then relates to the discussion above of how the *ren* and *du mai* are in resonance with *jing* and *shen*, respectively. If the *qiao mai* are seen as a development out of the *ren* and *du mai*, the initiation of movement in the Sea of Yin/*jing* and Sea of Yang/*shen* (as seen in Chapter 4), then they can be seen as relating to the *jing* and *shen* as they move and spiral through the body. This may help to further explain the master–couple pairing of the *yin qiao mai* and *ren mai*, and the *yang qiao mai* and *du mai*—the *ren mai* may be seen as the Sea of Jing, while the *yin qiao mai* may relate to the movement of *jing* through the body, and similar for the *du* and *yang qiao mai* in relation to *shen*. Thus they are reservoirs for each other. Further support is offered by Larre and Rochat de la Vallée: "the *qiao mai* follow the same pattern as the *du mai* and *ren mai* which are circling in a closed circulation. They are just a development of the *du mai* and *ren mai*" (1997, p. 204). This provides another direct connection between the *yin* and *yang qiao mai* (the movement of *jing* and *shen*) and the Marrow ("*jing* plus *shen*").

Another interesting correlation between the Marrow and the *qiao mai* can be seen by looking at *Su Wen* Chapter 17: "The bones are the palace of the marrow. If one cannot stand for prolonged periods or walk with stability, this means that the bones are about to be exhausted" (Ni 1995, p. 64). It can be inferred from this quotation that the Marrow is responsible for nourishing the Bones, and that the Marrow is therefore ultimately responsible for the ability to walk and stand—thus when there are problems with walking or standing, the Marrow is no longer nourishing the Bones. Interestingly, issues of gait are usually an indication of an imbalance in the *qiao mai* (the "Walker" vessels).

Further support of this connection between the *qiao mai* and the Marrow is also seen in that the Marrow pertains to the Kidneys, and the confluent points of both the *yin* and *yang qiao mai* are found on the Kidney and Bladder channels. Also, it has been said that "The Yang Motility vessel...enters the brain at Fengfu DU-16" (Deadman and Al-Khafaji 2005, p. 321); *fengfu* DU-16 is also a point of the Sea of Marrow.

Gall Bladder and *Dai Mai*: Returning to a State of Oneness

In pairing the extraordinary vessels and *fu*, the *dai mai* will clearly be the extraordinary vessel that corresponds to the Gall Bladder. While several correspondences between the *dai mai* and the Gall Bladder have already been examined in Chapter 3 (including the fact that the confluent point of the *dai mai* is located on the Gall Bladder channel— *zulinqi* GB-41), in this section I will further build on this discussion. In order to examine this connection in more depth, I will focus on the function of both the Gall Bladder and the *dai mai* to facilitate the return to Source and tonify the Kidneys/pre-heaven.

Previously in the history of Chinese medicine, there were some who thought that it was not possible to reach the Kidneys or the essence directly, and that the way to make this connection was through the Gall Bladder. As stated by Yuen:

The Gall Bladder is seen as the link between Post-Natal and Pre-Natal. Which is also the suggestion that some scholars have made within Chinese medicine, that, perhaps, without Eight Extra Channels, how the Chinese try to get into the level of *Jing*, was by working on the Gall Bladder... The idea is that, if you're going to tap into the Kidney, you tap into the Kidney through Gall Bladder. (2005, p. 31)

This is also seen with the *dai mai*, which binds the *ren*, *du* and *chong mai* at the level of the lower *dantian*, and through this connection may help one to return to the Source and pre-heaven state. Thus it may be that the *dai mai* and the Gall Bladder both play a role in connecting the post-heaven *qi* and essence of the Spleen with the pre-heaven *qi* and essence of the Kidneys at the Source.[2]

In looking at the Gall Bladder channel, we can see this process reflected on the hypochondriac region. Here one finds *riyue* GB-24, the front-*mu* point of the Gall Bladder, followed by a meeting point of the Gall Bladder channel with *zhangmen* LIV-13, the front-*mu* point of the Spleen and *hui*-meeting of the *zang*, as well as the starting point of the *dai mai*. This is then followed by *jingmen* GB-25, the front-*mu* point of the Kidneys. Here we can see a transition of accessing the Gall Bladder *qi* directly at *riyue* GB-24, which is then (perhaps) involved in connecting the post-heaven of the Spleen (accessed at *zhangmen* LIV-13) with the pre-heaven of the Kidneys (at *jingmen* GB-25), thereby

---

2 From this perspective, as long as this process is functioning correctly, the Kidneys should not become deficient, for post-heaven essence will continually replenish the pre-heaven essence—thus if there is Kidney deficiency, its root likely lies in the disruption of this mechanism.

directly nourishing and replenishing the Kidneys. It is also here that we find the starting point of the *dai mai* (again, at *zhangmen* LIV-13), which, in addition to connecting with *daimai* GB-26, *wushu* GB-27, and *weidao* GB-28, is said (according to some sources) to connect with *shenshu* BL-23 (back-*shu* of the Kidneys) and *mingmen* DU-4, as well as the *ren*, *du*, and *chong mai*, thus replenishing the pre-heaven of the Kidneys (and the quiescent state of the extraordinary vessels, as seen in the previous chapter; see Appendix).

Wei Mai and Bones: Integration and Protection

At this point, we have paired the *ren mai* with the Uterus, the *chong mai* with the Blood Vessels, the *du mai* with the Brain, the *qiao mai* with the Marrow, and the *dai mai* with the Gall Bladder. That leaves us with the *wei mai* and the Bones as the final pair to examine. In looking at the *wei mai* and Bones, at first glance it may seem as though there is very little correlation between this theoretical extraordinary vessel and extraordinary organ pairing. However, if we think of the *wei mai* as relating to protection and the creation of boundaries that connect ("link") the inside and the outside, and the Bones as protecting the internal organs and connecting and separating the inside and the outside (*zangfu* and primary channels, pre-heaven and post-heaven), then we can start to see a relation between the *wei mai* and Bones.[3]

---

3   The Bones may be thought of as the link between pre-heaven (as represented by Marrow/*jing*) and post-heaven (as represented by the tissues—tendons, blood vessels, muscles, and skin).

The Bones form the three cavities (pelvic, thoracic, and cranial) that protect the internal organs, creating boundaries that sustain the structure of the body as well as separate the *zangfu*, core, and interior from the primary channels, limbs, and exterior: "bones are the framework for the human body, like the trunk of a tree, and they stick to the flesh. They are also able to protect the *zang* on the interior, as in the thoracic cage, which is something like the hull of a ship" (Larre and Rochat de la Vallée 2003, p. 91). Similarly, the *wei mai* are also closely related to protection and connecting and separating the inside and the outside: "The two Linking vessels harmonize Interior–Exterior and Nutritive Qi–Defensive Qi" (Maciocia 2005, p. 828). The *wei mai* are also responsible for providing structure for the body, just as the Bones do. As stated by Larre and Rochat de la Vallée, the *yin* and *yang wei mai* "have a common function, to fasten and hold the body together" (1997, p. 215). Thus both the *wei mai* and the Bones function to give us stability here on Earth as individuated beings; they are primary bases of support.

The Bones are one of the main structures associated with the entering and exiting of *qi*: "Qi enters and exits from the bones on its way to and from the deep energetic layers of the body" (Maciocia 2005, p. 83). This "entering and exiting" of *qi* relates to horizontal integration, and is also a primary function of the *wei mai*: "commentators have said that the *yang wei mai* masters the exterior, and the movement towards the exterior, and the *yin wei* masters the interior and the movement towards the interior" (Larre and Rochat de la Vallée 1997, p. 214). Thus both the *wei mai* and the Bones may relate to the horizontal level of integration as represented by the entering and exiting of *qi*, connecting the interior and the exterior.

Interestingly, the *wei mai* are also said to start on the Kidney and Bladder channels (see Appendix). Just as both Marrow and Bones are said to pertain to the Kidneys, both the *qiao* and *wei mai* are said to start on these water channels. Just as the Marrow nourishes the Bones, it may be that the *qiao mai* nourish the *wei mai*, in this process of expanding out from the Source and connecting the inside and the outside, as seen in evolutionary unfolding of the extraordinary channels examined in the last chapter. Just as we saw above that the Marrow and the *qiao mai* both have an intimate relationship to the mobilization and movement of the essence from the Source to nourish the entire body, so too can it be seen that the *wei mai* and the Bones have an intimate relationship to integration, protection, and boundaries.

Further evidence of the connection between the *wei mai* and the Bones can be found by examining correspondences to Kidney *yang* and the Ministerial Fire. As examined in Chapter 2, Kidney *yang*, the *mingmen*, and the Pericardium–San Jiao systems are all said to belong to the Ministerial Fire. All three correspond to the right proximal pulse position, and have a relationship to regulating boundaries and intimate relationships—they both give us the strength to be independent beings at the level of humanity, and also provide the desire to dissolve our boundaries, to merge with and become "one" with another through relationship and physical intimacy.

Although I noted above that the *wei mai* have a relationship to the Kidneys and Bladder, as they are said to start on these channels, they also have a very close and intimate relationship with the Pericardium and San Jiao, as this is where their confluent points are located. As the *wei mai* are very closely related to boundaries, perhaps it can be said that they correspond relatively more to Kidney *yang* and the Ministerial Fire, similar to the Pericardium and San Jiao. Similarly, while both the Bones and the Marrow are said to correspond to the Kidneys, the Bones are also said to correspond more to Kidney *yang*, while Marrow corresponds to Kidney *yin*.[4] As stated by Larre and Rochat de la Vallée:

> The relationship between bones and marrow is that both are produced by the kidneys...there is a couple relationship between bones and marrow. They are like the soft and the hard, the *yin* and the *yang*, the interior and exterior... The expression "marrow and bone", sui gu (髓骨), shows the double power of the kidneys. Both *yin* and *yang* aspects of the kidneys are projected in the coupling of bones and marrow... (2003, p. 93)

This, then, would shed further light on the correspondences between the *qiao mai* and the Marrow, and the *wei mai* and the Bones—Marrow (and the *qiao mai*) can be seen to correspond relatively more to Kidney *yin*, to fluidity and the movement of the essence as it arises from the Source, while the Bones (and the *wei mai*) correspond more to Kidney *yang* and the Ministerial Fire, and thus provide the structure and container to direct the flow of movement of the *qiao mai* and the Marrow.

---

4   Further support of this is seen in that many herbal substances that are said to strengthen and repair Bones also tonify Kidney *yang*.

This, then, leaves us with a perfect one-to-one correspondence between the condensed extraordinary vessels (*ren mai, chong mai, du mai, qiao mai, wei mai,* and *dai mai*), and the six extraordinary organs, and the pairings may be posited as seen in Table 5.1:

Table 5.1 Pairing the Extraordinary Vessels and the Extraordinary Organs

Extraordinary vessel	Extraordinary organ
Ren mai	Uterus
Chong mai	Blood Vessels
Du mai	Brain
Qiao mai	Marrow
Wei mai	Bones
Dai mai	Gall Bladder

Summary of the Pairings

To summarize, we can see a strong relationship between the extraordinary vessels and the extraordinary organs. In this model, the *ren mai* and Uterus pertain to the lower *dantian* and relate to *jing*, the *du mai* and the Brain pertain to the upper *dantian* and relate to *shen*, and the *chong mai* and the *mai* pertain to the middle *dantian* and relate to *qi* and blood. These three pairs create the vertical axis of integration within the body, corresponding to the relatively pre-heaven, quiescent state of the Source as it first unfolds into the polarity of Heaven, Earth, and Humanity within the human body, as mirrored by the three *dantian*.

From this point we can see an expansion outward with the *qiao mai* and Marrow, both of which relate to the movement of the essence from the Source, as it expands out to nourish the internal organs and tissues (as well as the Bones and the *wei mai*). The *wei mai* and the Bones both assist in the process of integration and protection, creating the boundaries that simultaneously connect and separate the inside and the outside, and providing a structure and sense of integration for the movement of the essence. Finally, the Gall Bladder and *dai mai* assist in guiding the *qi* from post-heaven back to pre-heaven to nourish the lower *dantian*, Kidneys, and *ren, du* and *chong mai*. Pairing the extraordinary vessels and the extraordinary organs in this manner, it becomes easier to see their relation to creating and sustaining the individual human being.

Chapter 6

THE *YING QI* CYCLE AND THE EXTRAORDINARY ORGANS

In the last two chapters, we have explored a theoretical model that pairs the extraordinary vessels with the extraordinary organs in a one-to-one correspondence—similar to the way in which the *zangfu* are paired with the primary channels— as well as the way in which the extraordinary vessels may have a relation to the evolution of consciousness, as seen through the diurnal flow of the *ying qi* cycle. It becomes easier to see how the pairings of the extraordinary vessels and organs posited in the previous chapter fit together when examining the flow of the *ying qi* cycle. The *ying qi* cycle provides an elegant means to examine the associations of the paired extraordinary vessels and organs and their relation to vertical and horizontal integration, center and periphery, and the evolution of consciousness.

In following the unfoldment of the extraordinary vessels (as viewed through the *ying qi* cycle) we saw a clear reflection of the evolution of consciousness—the one breaking into two, into three, into the ten thousand things, allowing integration within oneself and connection to all else present at the level of humanity, and eventually transcending duality and returning to oneness to start the cycle again. In this chapter, we will take another journey through the *ying qi* cycle, to further expand on this model by examining the order of unfoldment of the paired extraordinary vessels and extraordinary organs. In combining these two models, it becomes apparent that the order in which the *ying qi* cycle theoretically accesses the extraordinary organs (as paired with the associated extraordinary vessel confluent points) also mirrors this process of the evolution of consciousness, and vertical and horizontal integration.

Lung through Small Intestine: Vertical Integration and Pre-Heaven

Starting in the Lung Channel of Hand Taiyin, corresponding to approximately 3–5am, the first confluent point we come to is *lieque* LU-7, confluent point of the *ren mai*. In the model proposed in the previous chapter, the *ren mai* is paired with the Uterus and *jing*, both of which correspond to the lower *dantian*. Thus we start at the quiescent state, the lower *dantian*, which is the source of the extraordinary vessels and pre-heaven. Within the extraordinary *fu*, the Uterus also corresponds to the most logical starting point, as it is the seat of the essence. As noted by Yuen, "if you were to follow a hierarchy of the Curious Organs, we would begin that hierarchy with the Uterus. The *Jing* Essence begins in the level of the Uterus" (2006, p. 69).

From the Lung channel, the *ying qi* continues through the Large Intestine and Stomach channels, until it flows into the Spleen channel and reaches *gongsun* SP-4, confluent point of the *chong mai*. At this point, the *ying qi* accesses the *chong mai* (within the extraordinary vessels), and therefore the Blood Vessels (within the extraordinary *fu*) and the middle *dantian*. Thus we move from the Uterus to the Blood Vessels, and from the lower to the middle *dantian*. Continuing on, the *ying qi* flows through the Heart channel and into the Small Intestine channel, until it reaches *houxi* SI-3, confluent point of the *du mai*—which in this model also corresponds to the Brain and the upper *dantian*.

Through these first six channels of the *ying qi* cycle (Lung–Small Intestine, 3am–3pm), we can see a clear unfoldment of the extraordinary vessels and organs corresponding to the three *dantian* and the vertical axis of integration within the body—starting from the lower *dantian*, Uterus, and *jing*, moving to the middle *dantian*, Blood Vessels, and *qi*, and finally reaching the upper *dantian*, Brain, and *shen* (see Table 6.1 below). This mirrors the process of internal alchemy, transforming *jing* into *qi* and *qi* into *shen*, and may be said to correspond to the vertical axis of integration and the quiescent state of the *ren, chong,* and *du mai*. This is the formation of the core of the body, corresponding primarily to pre-heaven and the Source. See Table 6.1 for an illustration of these correspondences.

Table 6.1 Correspondences of the Axis of Vertical Integration and Internal Alchemy

Energetic center	Extraordinary vessel	Extraordinary organ	Three treasures
Lower *dantian*	*Ren mai*	Uterus	*Jing*
Middle *dantian*	*Chong mai*	Blood Vessels	*Qi*
Upper *dantian*	*Du mai*	Brain	*Shen*

As was seen in Chapter 4, it is from this quiescent state of pre-heaven and vertical integration that manifestation, integration within self, and connection to everything else present at the level of humanity can occur, as represented by the activation of the *qiao* and *wei mai*. Therefore, the *qiao* and *wei mai* correspond relatively more to the state of post-heaven and horizontal integration within the extraordinary vessels. We can now continue along the *ying qi* cycle and, in observing their paired extraordinary *fu*, we will see this process mirrored once again.

Urinary Bladder–San Jiao: Horizontal Integration and Post-heaven

As the *ying qi* continues its diurnal flow, it exits the Small Intestine channel and enters the Urinary Bladder channel, beginning the second half of its daily cycle (corresponding to the time period 3pm–3am). Flowing through the Urinary Bladder channel, it arrives at *shenmai* BL-62, confluent point of the *yang qiao mai*, followed quickly by *zhaohai* K-6, confluent point of the *yin qiao mai*. As seen in Chapter 5, the *qiao mai* are paired with the Marrow; both the *qiao mai* and the Marrow share a relation to the movement of the essence out from the Source/lower *dantian*, and relate to global nourishment by the essence (especially nourishment of the Brain). Further, both the *qiao mai* and the Marrow may be said to have a strong correspondence to the legs (and motility and movement in general) and the ability to walk and move around and thus experience more at the level of humanity.

Besides the spinal cord and Brain, the long bones of the legs have the greatest concentration of Marrow within the body. If the Marrow and *qiao mai* have a strong correspondence to the legs, as well as to nourishing the

Brain (Sea of Marrow), perhaps they also relate to the connection between the feet and the Brain (macrocosmic Earth and Heaven). It is this connection between the Brain and the legs that allows each individual to walk around at the human level of reality.

This relation between the *qiao mai*, Marrow, and legs is significant and deserves further discussion. If both the *qiao mai* and the Marrow are seen as corresponding to the emergence of the post-heaven state from the Source/pre-heaven, then, within the extraordinary vessels and *fu*, they also correspond relatively more to horizontal integration and the periphery. Within the anatomy of the human body, the legs and arms also correspond more to horizontal integration and the periphery, relative to the trunk/core of the body. The legs allow the human being to move through the world and thus have a greater capacity for experiential awareness at the level of humanity—much as the *qiao mai* and Marrow relate to the movement of essence through the body, leading to the manifestation and nourishment of the individual human being.

Continuing along the *ying qi* cycle, we move into the Pericardium and San Jiao channels, where we reach *neiguan* P-6 and *waiguan* SJ-5—the confluent points of the *wei mai*, and therefore, by association, the Bones. As seen in the last chapter, the Marrow nourishes the Bones, just as the *qiao mai* may be said to nourish the *wei mai*, while the Bones and the *wei mai* provide the structure and stability to allow for the smooth flow of the essence (*qiao mai* and Marrow) through the body.

If the *qiao mai* and Marrow are seen as being in correspondence with the legs, perhaps the *wei mai* and Bones may be seen as being in correspondence with the arms. The *qiao mai* pertain relatively more to the legs as they are "walker" vessels and their confluent points are on the foot *taiyang* and foot *shaoyin* channels, while the *wei mai* may pertain more to the arms as they are the "linking" vessels, and their confluent points are on the hand *shaoyang* and hand *jueyin* channels. It is the hands and arms that allow us to truly connect and link to everything else around us, and thus correspond to the level of humanity.

This association is also seen in some Daoist traditions—according to Deng Ming-Dao, the *yang wei mai* "travel bilaterally along the back of each arm, around the tip of the middle fingers, along the inside of the middle fingers to the point *laogong*," while the *yin wei mai* travel "[f]rom the *laogong* point of the palm…along the inside of each arm, curve across the pectoral muscles, descend through the nipples, and connect with the renmei via a brief trip along the *daimei*" (1990, pp. 93–94). Therefore, *laogong* P-8 is said to be, in this Daoist tradition, a meeting point of the *yin wei mai* and *yang wei mai*. This then lends even further evidence of the relationship between the arms and the *wei mai*, for the arms correspond to the level of humanity, and *laogong* P-8—in the center of the palms—is the point where one exchanges *qi* with the level of humanity. Although it is the legs and feet that connect to Earth and allow each individual to move through the world, it is the arms and hands that allow each individual to truly connect ("link") to everything else present at the level of humanity—as humans, we wave to each other, shake and hold hands, hug and embrace, and touch to experience and connect to the world around us.

Similarly, it is the Bones that create channels for the Marrow to flow through, linking the flow of essence throughout the body and providing the structure of connection and integration. The Bones also participate in the entering and exiting of *qi*, and thereby assist in the connection between oneself and everything else present at the level of humanity. Further, the arms and hands are relatively more "bony" than the legs or other parts of the body—the arms do not have nearly the concentration of Marrow of the legs, nor do they have as much musculature. Thus, the *wei mai* and Bones have a close association to the arms and hands, and all three share correspondences to horizontal integration and the periphery, as well as functioning to link us to others and the world around us.

Here we can see a beautiful resonance—the *ren*, *chong*, and *du mai*, as well as the Uterus, *mai*, and Brain, correspond to the trinities of the three *dantian* and the three treasures that form the vertical axis of integration within the body, connecting Heaven, Earth, and Humanity, above and below. They are the three aspects of the *taiji*, the Supreme Polarity of *yin*, *yang*, and the pivot between; thus they are three, yet one. They correspond to the core of the body and the relatively pre-heaven state, and are the "nuclear" extraordinary vessels. It is this axis of vertical integration/pre-heaven that allows one to experience horizontal axis of integration, connecting the inside and the outside, connecting with all else present at the level of humanity. The *qiao* and *wei mai* are the "peripheral" extraordinary vessels and are in a state of duality, having both *yin* and *yang* channels, and they correspond relatively more to the duality of the two legs and two arms. Pre-heaven is a state of unity; post-heaven is a state of duality.

Gall Bladder–Liver: Transcendence and the Return to Unity

Finally, as the *ying qi* flows into the Gall Bladder channel and reaches *zulinqi* GB-41, the *dai mai* and Gall Bladder are accessed and there is the opportunity for balance between these processes of vertical and horizontal integration, allowing one to transcend duality, reach a state of wholeness, and return to the Source to start a new cycle. As we examined in previous chapters, the *dai mai* and Gall Bladder both assist in connecting back to the pre-heaven of the Kidneys, Uterus, and lower *dantian*, as well as the quiescent state of the extraordinary vessels, bringing the post-heaven essence back to nourish pre-heaven and preparing to start the cycle again the next day. This corresponds to the movement from the greatest exterior and expanded state back to the deepest interior.

Clearly, the *dai mai* and Gall Bladder play a role in rendering the *yin* and *yang* aspects of being into a unified whole and allow one to start a new cycle again the next day. This ability and function of both the *dai mai* and the Gall Bladder to transcend duality and facilitate the return to Source on a daily basis is significant. This is a challenging point of transition that occurs not only within the daily flow of the *ying qi* through the primary channels, but also within the evolution of consciousness as mirrored by the daily unfoldment of the extraordinary vessels and *fu*, and relates to the drive towards transcendence. Perhaps it is also for this reason that the Gall Bladder is associated with courage—it takes courage to maintain the dynamic tension between vertical and horizontal integration, and to make the transition from the greatest exterior back to the deepest interior, from a state of duality to a state of unity, for it is a form of death and rebirth.

This movement from the exterior back to the interior, and from duality to a state of unity, is also demonstrated in the place of the Gall Bladder as the only organ which is considered both an extraordinary organ and one of the

12 *zangfu.* As seen previously, the 12 primary channels and the *zangfu* relate to the mundane aspects of life and duality, while the extraordinary vessels and the extraordinary organs relate more to spiritual aspects of being, unity, and the evolution of consciousness. The Gall Bladder, which is both one of the *zangfu* and one of the six extraordinary *fu*, helps in bridging this movement from the mundane to the spiritual, from duality back to oneness.

Further, if the *qiao mai* and the Marrow, and *wei mai* and the Bones, are said to correspond to the legs and arms, respectively, then perhaps the *dai mai* and Gall Bladder can be said to correspond to the head. In the *Ode of the Obstructed River* are discussed the "Eight Therapeutic Methods" of using the confluent points of the extraordinary meridians to treat specific areas and symptoms. Here *zulinqi* GB-41 is indicated for disorders of the eyes, which may offer confirmation of the influence of the *dai mai* at the level of the upper *dantian* and head region (as cited in Deadman and Al-Khafaji 2005). Also, in looking at the pathway of the Gall Bladder channel, we see that it traces back and forth across the top, sides, and back of the head, demonstrating a strong relationship and sphere of impact of the Gall Bladder on the Brain, upper *dantian*, and head as a whole. In fact, the Gall Bladder channel has 20 points, nearly half the points of the channel, located on the head—many more than any other channel. Further, as seen above, the Gall Bladder is a bridge between duality and oneness—just as the head is considered both an extremity and part of the core of the body.

Just as the legs and arms are in a state of duality (as are the *qiao* and *wei mai*), the head is a singular peripheral extremity. Therefore, in the second half of the *ying qi* cycle, there is reflected once again the movement from the lower *dantian*, to the middle *dantian*, to the upper *dantian*. The *qiao mai* and Marrow correspond to the legs (as well as grounding and movement), which can be seen as an extension out from the lower *dantian*, while the *wei mai* and Bones have correspondences to the arms (as well as integration and boundaries), which can be seen as an extension out from the middle *dantian*. The *dai mai* and Gall Bladder, relating to transcendence and the return to oneness, correspond to the head and the upper *dantian*. The head shares aspects of both core and periphery—thus it is a meeting place of duality and unity, and the place where one connects to Heaven (oneness) while present at the level of manifestation (duality). This also speaks to the above discussion of the *dai mai* and Gall Bladder facilitating the return to oneness, moving from duality (legs and arms, Earth and Humanity) back to unity (the head, upper *dantian*, and Heaven). See Table 6.2 for a graphic illustration of these relationships.

Further evidence that the first half of the *ying qi* cycle corresponds to the vertical axis, and the second half of the *ying qi* cycle corresponds to the horizontal axis, is seen in the distribution of the extraordinary vessel confluent points. There are three extraordinary vessels (*ren, chong,* and *du mai*) accessed in the first half of the *ying qi* cycle, and these three correspond to the three *dantian* and the vertical axis. And there are five extraordinary vessels (*yin* and *yang qiao mai, yin* and *yang wei mai,* and the *dai mai*) accessed in the second half of the *ying qi* cycle, and these five relate more to the horizontal axis. Recall that the numbers three and five correspond to vertical and horizontal, respectively, as seen previously in relationship to the three *dantian* (vertical) and the five *zangfu* (horizontal).

Table 6.2 The Ying Qi Cycle and Evolutionary Unfoldment

Ying qi cycle	Confluent points	Extraordinary vessel	Extraordinary *fu*	Vertical and horizontal associations
LU–LI	LU-7	*Ren mai*	Uterus	Lower *dantian/Jing*
SP–ST	SP-4	*Chong mai*	Vessels/*mai*	Middle *dantian/Qi*
HE–SI	SI-3	*Du mai*	Brain	Upper *dantian/Shen*
K–BL	BL-62, K-6	*Qiao mai*	Marrow	Legs and feet/Movement
P–SJ	P-6, SJ-5	*Wei mai*	Bones	Arms and hands/Integration
LIV–GB	GB-41	*Dai mai*	Gall Bladder	Head/Transcendence

Chapter 7

PAIRING THE EXTRAORDINARY VESSELS WITH THE PRIMARY CHANNELS AND *ZANGFU*

In this chapter I will explore various connections between the primary channels/*zangfu* and the extraordinary vessels, further developing this theoretical model and examining ways in which the extraordinary vessels and primary channels/*zangfu* may have a direct correspondence to each other. To develop this perspective, I will examine anatomical, functional, and relational correspondences between the extraordinary vessels and the primary channels and *zangfu*, continuing to utilize the structure of the horary clock as the primary framework for exploration. As already seen, there is a specific distribution of the extraordinary vessel confluent points among the primary channels; in fact, there is a perfect, one-to-one distribution between each extraordinary vessel and each *zangfu*/primary channel pair (see Table 7.1).

Table 7.1 Pairing the Extraordinary Vessels and the Primary Channels

Primary channels and *zangfu*	Confluent points	Extraordinary vessel
Lung–Large Intestine	*Lieque* LU-7	*Ren mai*
Spleen–Stomach	*Gongsun* SP-4	*Chong mai*
Heart–Small Intestine	*Houxi* SI-3	*Du mai*
Kidney–Urinary Bladder	*Zhaohai* K-6, *Shenmai* BL-62	*Qiao mai*
Pericardium–San Jiao	*Neiguan* P-6, *Waiguan* SJ-5	*Wei mai*
Liver–Gall Bladder	*Zulinqi* GB-41	*Dai mai*

General Support

Before we examine the pairings individually, it will be useful to review some of the general information regarding the extraordinary vessels and the connections to their respective primary channels and *zangfu*. To start with, it has been said that one indication for utilizing an extraordinary vessel treatment strategy is when there is a disorder in the *zangfu* of the primary channel where its confluent point is located—that is, using the *ren mai* (whose confluent point is *lieque* LU-7) for all Lung issues and imbalances. As stated by Pirog in his discussion of the *ren mai*:

> [T]he symptoms of the meridian on which the master point is located must be incorporated into the list of indications for the associated extraordinary vessel.

In this case, the ren mai is linked to the lung meridian through Lu 7. Because of this connection, the lung function is more closely related to the ren mai than to any other extraordinary vessel. We must therefore include the full variety of lung patterns…as potential indications for ren mai treatment. (1996, p. 170)

This suggests that there is a strong association between each extraordinary vessel and the primary channel where its confluent point is located (as well as the *zangfu* of that primary channel). It further suggests that there is an important, underlying connection between the extraordinary vessel and its associated primary channel and *zangfu* pair.

It is also of note that, of the eight confluent points, four of them (*lieque* LU-7, *gongsun* SP-4, *neiguan* P-6, and *waiguan* SJ-5) are also the *luo*-connecting points of the primary channel on which they are found. This is significant, as *luo*-connecting points are one of the primary distal places along the channel where the *yin* and *yang* aspects of each pair of primary channels and *zangfu* meet and connect to each other. This suggests that there may be an important relationship between these confluent points (and their associated extraordinary vessel) and the connection between the interior–exterior related primary channels where they are located. For example, the *ren mai* likely has correlations to the Large Intestine as well as the Lung, and perhaps even to the connection *between* the Lung and the Large Intestine, given the nature of *lieque* LU-7 as both the confluent point of the *ren mai* and the *luo*-connecting point of the Lung channel.

This overlap may also shed further light on the 27th Difficult Issue: "Here [in the organism], when the network-vessels are filled to overflowing, none of the [main] conduits could seize any [of their contents, and it is only then that the surplus contents of these vessels flow into the single-conduit {i.e. extraordinary} vessels]" (Unschuld 1986, p. 322). If it is the extraordinary vessels that are responsible for absorbing surplus from the *luo*-connecting (i.e. network) channels, it then becomes clear why several of the extraordinary vessel confluent points overlap with *luo*-connecting points. In needling that point, one is simultaneously addressing the imbalance in the *luo* while accessing an extraordinary vessel that may be able to help regulate the *luo*. And, as *luo*-connecting points are the connection between interior–exterior paired primary channels, the extraordinary vessels may directly regulate the *luo* of the primary channels and *zangfu* where their confluent points are found.

Of the remaining four confluent points, it is of note that *zulinqi* GB-41 is the exit point of the Gall Bladder channel, and thus the point where the Gall Bladder channel diverges to connect with the Liver channel—suggesting that the *dai mai* may have a correspondence to the Liver as well as the Gall Bladder (and possibly to the connection between them). Lastly, not only are the confluent points of the *qiao mai* (*zhaohai* K-6 and *shenmai* BL-62) said to be the starting points of the *yin* and *yang qiao mai*, respectively, clearly demonstrating a close connection between these extraordinary vessels and their associated primary channels and *zangfu*, but the *qiao mai* themselves have often been likened to *luo* vessels of the Kidney and Bladder channels— the significance of this will be examined later on in more depth.

The Quiescent State and the First Six Primary Channels

In order to examine the individual relationship of each extraordinary vessel to its associated primary channel pair, we will begin by looking at the groupings of the first half of the horary clock (the time period from 3am to 3pm, corresponding to Lung–Large Intestine, Stomach–Spleen, and Heart–Small Intestine) and their relationship to the extraordinary vessels that form the quiescent state (*ren mai*, *chong mai*, and *du mai*).

In this model, the Lungs and Large Intestine (*zangfu* and primary channels) correspond to the *ren mai*. As mentioned above, *lieque* LU-7 is both the confluent point of the *ren mai* and the *luo*-connecting point of the Lung channel, suggesting a possible relationship between the *ren mai* and the connection between the Lung and Large Intestine channels. Beyond this, there are several other strong correspondences between anatomical and functional aspects of the *ren mai* to these Metal channels and organs.

For starters, the Lungs are said to house the *po*, the corporeal soul. This is the relatively more physical, material, *yin* aspect of the *shen*. Similarly, the *ren mai* pertains more to the physical, material, *yin* aspects of being, and corresponds very closely to the *jing*-essence. The *ren mai* is called the Sea of Yin, yet (as noted in earlier chapters) it may also be called the Sea of *Jing* when examining the *ren*, *chong*, and *du mai* in relation to the three treasures. And there is an intimate connection between the *po* and the *jing*-essence, as noted by Maciocia:

> The entering and exiting of Qi are also controlled by the Corporeal Soul (*Po*), which is in charge of the entering

and exiting of the Essence (*Jing*). In other words, the Corporeal Soul and the Essence are closely coordinated and the Corporeal Soul is sometimes described as the "entering and exiting of the Essence". For this reason, the Corporeal Soul contributes to all physiological activities. (2005, pp. 80–81)

This suggests a strong link between the Lungs and the *ren mai*, as relates to the *jing* and the *po*. The *po* is the most physical/material aspect of the *shen*, and the *jing*-essence is the material/physical substance of experiential reality; together, the *po* and the *jing* are regulated by the *ren mai* and the Lungs.

A further correspondence, related to this resonance between the *po* (Lungs) and the *jing* (*ren mai*), is seen in the way in which both the *ren mai* and the Lungs relate to the process of embodiment, of taking on "the burden of being human" and existing in the world at this level. As stated by Miriam Lee:

> As the lung qi works physically in the body against the force of gravity to hold up tears, etc., so too lung qi on an emotional or soul level holds up the spirit against the gravity of our struggle to survive in the world. When the lung qi is low, that knowledge of how to live becomes weaker and may be lost. When this soul goes, the person's will to live is gone. (1992, p. 41)

This sentiment is echoed when we examine the etymology of the Chinese character for "*ren*":

...to bear the burden of being human, which is for instance, to be able to take charge and cope at each level of human life: to cope with each situation, to endure, to withstand, and to be able to resist attack. At the same time this idea of being able to withstand is softened by the notion of following the natural way. It is coping, not by confrontation, but allowing. (Larre and Rochat de la Vallée 1997, p. 85)

Therefore, both the *ren mai* and the Lungs may relate to the process of embodiment, of taking on the charge of being human and all that it entails.

Further, to examine it from an anatomical perspective, part of the Lung channel pathway is in close relation to the *ren mai*. As summarized by Pirog:

Recall that the internal course of the lung meridian, which begins at RM 12, descends down the ren mai to the lower abdomen, and reascends up the ren mai to RM 17 before surfacing at Lu 1... The lung meridian therefore shares some of its internal trajectory with the ren mai. (1996, p. 168)

Thus, even beyond the close relationships demonstrated by their connections to the *po* and the *jing*, and the process of embodiment, the *ren mai* and the Lung channel have confluence in their energetic pathways as well.

The *Chong Mai* and the Spleen and Stomach

Next we can examine some of the correspondences between the *chong mai* and the Stomach and Spleen. As noted above, *gongsun* SP-4 is the confluent point of the *chong mai* and the *luo*-connecting point of the Spleen channel, and thus may share in this connection between the Spleen and Stomach. Beyond this, there are numerous other relationships between the *chong mai* and the Spleen and Stomach systems.

Anatomically, the *chong mai* shares many points with the Kidney channel; it also resonates functionally with the Kidneys (see Appendix).[1] However, it also has numerous connections to the Spleen and Stomach channels. As stated in the *Nan Jing* (Classic of Difficult Issues), "The throughway vessel originates from the *ch'i-ch'ung* [hole] {*qichong* ST-30}, parallels the foot-yang-brilliance-conduit, ascends near the navel, and reaches the chest, where it dissipates" (Unschuld 1986, p. 327). And as noted in the *Su Wen* (Plain Questions), Chapter 60: "In disorders of the chong/vitality channel, the qi will rebel upward, causing acute abdominal pain and contracture" (Ni 1995, p. 209).

Li Shi Zhen further summarizes:

> Surfacing and externalizing, it arises at Qi Thoroughfare (ST-30)... Here, it travels alongside and between the

---

1   It is important to note that the three extraordinary vessels that form the quiescent state (*ren*, *chong*, and *du mai*) all have a deep, intimate relationship to the lower *dantian* and the Kidneys. Thus it is not surprising that they would each have strong connections to the Kidneys as well as their respective *zangfu* and primary channels as proposed in this book. It is even plausible that they are thereby able to connect the Kidneys with their respective *zangfu* (e.g. the *chong mai* helps to connect the Kidneys with the Spleen and Stomach). For example, see Chase and Shima: "The *chong* vessel may be understood as the axis by which the stomach channel communicates earthly qi, and the kidney channel communicates heavenly qi, throughout the body" (2010, p. 237). This will be touched on again later on.

two channels of the foot yang brightness and lesser yin and proceeds along the abdomen, traveling upward to the pubic bone. (The foot yang brightness [channel] is located two *cun* from the midline of the abdomen; the foot lesser yin [channel] is located five *fen* from the midline of the abdomen; the trajectory of the *chong* vessel travels between these two vessels...) (Chase and Shima 2010, p. 123)

Li later continues, quoting [Wang] Qi-Xuan: "'Because the *chong* vessel lies beneath the spleen [channel], it is said that the *chong* is located beneath,' and it is called Greater Yin" (Chase and Shima 2010, p. 125). This demonstrates a strong connection between the *chong mai* and the Spleen and Stomach systems and a confluence in their channel pathways. Continuing from the anatomical perspective, it is also of note that the *chong mai* is said to travel around the mouth, which is the sense organ corresponding to the Spleen and Stomach.

It is also important to note that the *chong mai* is known as the Sea of the Five *Zang* and the Six *Fu*, as well as the Sea of the 12 Channels. According to the *Jia Yi Jing* (The Systematic Classic of Acupuncture and Moxibustion): "The penetrating vessel is the sea of the five viscera and the six bowels. The five viscera and six bowels are dependent on it for nourishment" (Mi 2004, p. 55). This is possibly related to its nature as the pivot between the fundamental polarity of *yin* and *yang* in the channel system, as represented by the *ren* and *du mai*. Similarly, the Spleen and Stomach are said to be the Sea of the *Zangfu* and are also often referred to as the pivot within the internal organ system. For this reason, the Spleen and Stomach are often depicted as the *taiji* symbol, as the central pivot of *yin* and *yang* that are basis of the other *zangfu*.

As summarized by Larre and Rochat de la Vallée, in examining how both the *chong mai* and the Stomach are said to be the Sea of the five *zang* and the six *fu*:

> We can see here the strong relationship between the *chong mai* and the stomach meridian, which work together. The stomach is able to continually renew the essences through digestion and assimilation, but it is unable to regulate the distribution of *qi* and essences on its own. The *chong mai* represents the pattern of organisation for the distribution. (1997, p. 115)

The classical texts and earlier commentators have also noted this confluence between the *chong mai* and the Stomach and Spleen. As stated in the *Su Wen* (Plain Questions), Chapter 44:

> Yangming is the source of nourishment for all the zang fu viscera. Only with this nourishment can the tendons, bones, and joints be lubricated. The chong/ vitality channel is considered the reservoir of the twelve main meridians. It is responsible for the permeability of nutrients throughout the body and into the muscles. It works together with the yangming in this function. The yangming/stomach can be said to be the primary channel that is responsible for this. (Ni 1995, pp. 164–165)

And by Zhang Jing-Yue:

[T]he yang brightness is the sea of the five viscera and six receptacles, while the *chong* is the sea of the channels and vessels. Of these, one is yin and one is yang, but between them, they constitute the totality [of all the channels]. (Cited in Chase and Shima 2010, pp. 250–251)

These statements offer further support to the perspective that the Spleen and Stomach (organs and channels) share a direct correspondence with the *chong mai*.

Above we examined the relationship between the *ren mai* as the Sea of *Jing* to the Lungs and the *po*. Within the paradigm of the three treasures, the *chong mai* may also be called the Sea of *Qi*, and within the correspondences between the extraordinary vessels and the extraordinary organs it may be said to relate to the Blood Vessels, as seen in Chapter 5. This, then, has an interesting correspondence to the function of the Spleen and Stomach to produce *qi* and blood, as well as the function of the Spleen to hold the blood in the vessels.

The *Du Mai* and the Heart and Small Intestine

The third pairing we will examine in this section is the relationship between the *du mai* and the Heart and Small Intestine systems. As you may have noticed above in the discussion on general support, *houxi* SI-3 was the only confluent point not mentioned as having some direct connection to the paired channels and *zangfu*. Although *houxi* SI-3 is not a *luo*-connecting point or an exit point, there is another, more direct connection linking the *du mai* to the Heart and to Heart function. The course of the *du mai* itself passes through the Heart, which is one of the only direct connections between an extraordinary vessel and a *zangfu* organ (see Appendix). As stated in the *Su Wen* (Plain Questions), Chapter 60, "The [*du*] channel crosses the umbilicus, goes up *through the heart* into the throat and around the mouth, stopping below the eyes" (Ni 1995, p. 209; emphasis added). Also, as stated in the *Jia Yi Jing* (The Systematic Classic):

> The branch [of the governing vessel] which travels straight upward from the lower abdomen runs through the center of the umbilicus, penetrates the heart, and enters the throat… If (the governing vessel) becomes diseased, there will be a surging ascension (of qi) from the lower abdomen into the heart and resultant (heart) pain and inability to defecate or urinate. (Mi 2004, p. 56)

The course of the *du mai* also connects directly to the Kidneys. As stated in the *Su Wen* (Plain Questions), Chapter 60:

> It then travels around the anal area and branches again through the thigh, where it connects with the foot shaoyin/kidney channel. It combines with the luo/ collateral of foot taiyang and foot shaoyin to converge in the buttocks. It travels upward from there, penetrating the spine and finally connecting with the kidneys. (Ni 1995, p. 209)

This lends further support to the theory that the *du mai* has a role in connecting the Heart and Kidneys to each other.

These connections demonstrate that there exists a relatively direct relationship between the *du mai* and the Heart and Small Intestine primary channels and *zangfu*.

Besides these anatomical connections linking the *du mai* to the Heart and Small Intestine, there are a number of functional and relational correspondences between this extraordinary vessel and this *zangfu* and primary channel system. As noted previously, although the *du mai* is often called the Sea of Yang, it may also be called the Sea of *Shen* from the perspective of the three treasures and the three *dantian*. Within this theoretical model, the *du mai* is seen as having an intimate relationship to the three *dantian* and the movement of *shen* between these centers of consciousness. Interestingly, the three *dantian* roughly correspond anatomically to the locations of the Small Intestine, Heart, and Brain. Related to this, it is noteworthy that the *du mai* is traditionally used to treat many disorders related to the *shen*, which is said (according to some sources) to reside in the Heart. Thus we see a clear correspondence between the Heart and Small Intestine systems and the *du mai*, as relates to the *shen*.

Along these lines, it is of note that *guan yuan* RN-4, one of the primary acupuncture points associated with the lower *dantian*, is also the front-*mu* point of the Small Intestine. Continuing further, the location of the lower *dantian* corresponds anatomically to the Uterus (which, in this model, is paired with the *ren mai*) in women and the Small Intestine (which is paired with the *du mai*) in men. Therefore, although the lower *dantian* is the source of *ren mai*, *chong mai*, and *du mai*, which are three yet one, it may be associated slightly more with the primary *yin* meridian (*ren mai*) for women and the primary *yang* meridian (*du mai*) for men through these correspondences.

The Heart and Small Intestine are the Emperor Fire, as compared with the Minister Fire of the Pericardium and San Jiao. The Emperor Fire corresponds relatively more to the vertical connection between Heaven, Earth, and Humanity, while the Ministerial Fire corresponds more to the horizontal connection between the inside and outside, and self and other. Similarly, the *du mai* relates more to vertical integration and connection, while the *wei mai*, Pericardium, and San Jiao are relatively more associated with horizontal integration. We also see this correspondence to vertical integration reflected in the first half of the *ying qi* cycle, and it is in this first half that we find both the Emperor Fire of the Heart–Small Intestine system and the confluent point of the *du mai*.

Lastly, the *du mai* also has a branch that connects directly to the tongue, which is the sense organ associated with the Heart and Small Intestine. As stated in the *Jia Yi Jing* (The Systematic Classic):

> Loss of Voice Gate (*Yin Men*) [Du 15] is also known as Tongue's Horizontal (*She Heng*) and Tongue Repression (She Yan) and is located on the nape of the neck in a depression in the hairline. It enters to connect with the root of the tongue and is a meeting point of the governing vessel and the yang linking vessel. (Mi 2004, p. 80)

And as noted in the footnote, "This implies that the governing vessel starts from this point to connect to the root of the tongue" (p. 113). Thus there is ample evidence of a very close relationship between the *du mai* and the Heart and Small Intestine systems.

Vertical Integration: Heaven, Earth, and Humanity

In summary, there is evidence of a deeper relationship between the first three pairs of interiorly–exteriorly related primary channels and *zangfu* and the three extraordinary vessels that form the quiescent state. There are numerous correlations suggesting a direct relationship between the Lungs/Large Intestine and the *ren mai*, the Spleen/ Stomach and the *chong mai*, and the Heart/Small Intestine and the *du mai* when the three pairings are examined individually. Alternatively, we can also look at these three systems as a whole—as the *ren–chong–du mai* are said to be three branches of one vessel—to reveal further insight into the relationship between these extraordinary vessels and their corresponding primary channels/*zangfu*.

One of the most important correspondences of these two separate systems—*ren–chong–du mai* and Lungs– Spleen–Heart—is the connection they share to the vertical axis and Daoist conceptions of cosmogenesis. The vertical axis corresponds not only to the manifestation and unfoldment of the oneness into the triad of Heaven, Earth, and Humanity, but also to the transcendence of duality and the return to oneness. We can see these two separate processes both represented in the first half of the *ying qi* cycle. On the one hand, we see the process of manifestation, as represented by the movement from the Lungs to the Spleen to the Heart (when we follow the flow of the *ying qi* cycle through the first six primary channels of the horary clock). Within these three *zang*, the Lungs correspond to Heaven above, the Spleen corresponds to Earth, and the Heart corresponds to Humanity.

This can be seen by examining the anatomical placement of these three organs as a system—the Lungs correspond to Heaven above, the Spleen and Stomach correspond to Earth, and the Heart, at the level of Humanity, is situated in the middle between the Spleen/Stomach system below and the Lungs above. Also notice the relationship of their associated sense organs—as stated by He-Shang Gong: "Dark refers to Heaven. In man, this means the nose, which links us with Heaven. Womb [female] refers to Earth. In man, this means the mouth, which links us to earth" (as cited in Chase and Shima 2010, p. 66). Therefore, the Lungs (as the nose is the flowering of the Lungs) are a reflection of Heaven, and the Spleen (as the mouth is the flowering of the Spleen) is a reflection of Earth. In various practices of *qigong*, meditation, and internal alchemy, one places the tongue (the flowering of the Heart) against the roof of the mouth, thereby helping to connect Heaven above (the nose/Lungs) with Earth below (the mouth/Spleen), as well as connecting the *du mai* (Heaven/*yang*) with the *ren mai* (Earth/*yin*). Thus, within the first half of the *ying qi* cycle through the primary channels, we have the movement from Heaven (Lungs) to Earth (Spleen) to Humanity (Heart), which corresponds to the process of manifestation in the evolution of consciousness—the process of the *dao* giving birth to one, to two, to three.

On the other hand, when looking at the relationship of the extraordinary vessels to the first half of the *ying qi* cycle, we have the process of internal alchemy, of transcending duality to reconnect with the oneness, as represented by the movement from the *ren mai* (lower *dantian/jing*-essence/ Uterus) to the *chong mai* (middle *dantian/qi/mai*) to the *du mai* (upper *dantian/shen*/Brain). This is a reflection of the transformation of *jing* to *qi* and *qi* to *shen*, as well as a movement from Earth to Humanity to Heaven, and is an ascension along the *zhong mai* (Central Channel) or *taiji* pole. Interestingly, this may shed further light on Luo Dong-Yi's discussion of the "grand thoroughfare." As stated by Chase and Shima:

> One common theme in Luo's use of the term is that the grand thoroughfare is invariably associated with the transmission of prenatal qi…the direction of this transmission is always upward from below… Luo Dong-Yi explains that the grand thoroughfare may also be used as a collective term for the *chong*, *ren*, and *du* vessels. (2010, pp. 318–319)

This difference between the primary channels and extraordinary vessels is fitting, as it is the *zangfu* and primary channels that correspond more to the day-to-day activity associated with manifestation and living in the mundane world at the level of humanity, whereas it is the extraordinary vessels that help to take us beyond the mundane, to reconnect to the Source and remember where we come from. See Table 7.2 for further illustration of these processes.

Table 7.2 The Ying Qi Cycle and the Processes
of Manifestation and Transcendence

Ying qi cycle	Zangfu	Process of manifestation	Extraordinary vessel	Process of transcendence
LU–LI	Lung	Heaven (一)	*Ren mai*	Earth/lower *dantian*
ST–SP	Spleen	Earth (二)	*Chong mai*	Humanity/ middle *dantian*
HE–SI	Heart	Humanity (三)	*Du mai*	Heaven/upper *dantian*

The *Qiao Mai* and the Kidneys and Bladder System

Turning to the second half of the horary clock, we come to the Kidney and Urinary Bladder primary channels and *zangfu*, which are paired with the *qiao mai* in this theoretical model. In the horary clock, these primary channels correspond to the time period 3–7pm; as the *ying qi* flows through these channels, it passes the confluent points of the *yang qiao mai* (*shenmai* BL-62) and the *yin qiao mai* (*zhaohai* K-6). As noted previously, the confluent points of the *qiao mai* are also the starting points of these extraordinary vessels, thus demonstrating a very close connection of the *yang qiao mai* with the Bladder channel and the *yin qiao mai* with the Kidney channel. As stated in the *Ling Shu* (Spiritual Pivot):

> The Yin Anklebone Channel separates from the Minor Yin and begins behind Blazing Valley [*rangu* KD-2; modern descriptions say that it starts from *zhaohai* KD-6]... It enters the cheekbones, subordinates the

inner corner of the eye, and joins with the Major Yang, Bladder Channel, and the Yang Anklebone Channel and travels up. When the qi move mutually and together, it will result in nourishing the eyes. When the qi does not prosper, it will result in the eyes not closing. (Wu 1993, p. 88)

The *qiao mai* literally "branch off" from the Kidney and Bladder primary channels, and for this reason have even been likened to *luo*-connecting channels of the Kidney and Bladder. As summarized by John Pirog:

> The yin and yang qiao mai are the only two extraordinary vessels that have master points which physically intersect with their pathways. The master points, in fact, are actually the starting points for these two vessels: Ki 6 for yin qiao mai and UB 62 for yang qiao mai. This results in a channel structure that is reminiscent of that of the luo vessels, with the two vessels branching directly out of their "home" meridians. This connection creates a close affinity between yin and yang qiao mai and the meridians they branch from. (1996, p. 178)

The comparisons made between the *qiao mai* and *luo* vessels is quite significant, given that four of the other confluent points are also the *luo*-connecting points of their respective primary channels, as noted above. We see this theme expanded when examining the *qiao mai* and the Kidney and Bladder channels, in relation to the intersection of *yin* and *yang*. As stated in the *Ling Shu* (Spiritual Pivot):

The Leg Major Yang has a penetration at the nape of the neck which enters into the brain... This penetration enters the brain at the separation of the Yin Anklebone Channel and the Yang Anklebone Channel, for yin and yang intersect mutually, so that yang enters yin and yin comes out of yang with a crossing at the medial corner of the eye. When the yang qi is full, it causes the eyes to glare and remain open. When the yin qi is full, it causes the eyes to close. (Wu 1993, p. 99)

Here again we see the close relation and intersection of the *qiao mai* with the Bladder channel, as well as their close relationship to the coming together and intersecting of *yin* and *yang*. This theme is continued in Larre and Rochat de la Vallée, citing Zhang Zicong:

Tai yang and shao yin of the foot are the source from which blood and qi, yin and yang are originally produced. Yin qiao mai and yang qiao mai master the free communication of yin and yang. Blood and qi from below rise and have an exchange and mutual connection at the eyes. (1997, p. 186)

Another significant association between the Kidney–Bladder system and the *qiao mai* is their relationship to Marrow (which is the extraordinary organ associated with the *qiao mai*, in this system), and specifically the Sea of Marrow (the Brain). The Marrow corresponds to the Kidneys and Bladder, and it is from the Kidneys that the *jing*-essence transforms into Marrow and moves through the body to nourish and sustain the organism. Specifically, the *jing*-essence descends from between the

Kidneys to the perineum, where it enters the tip of the tailbone, rises up through the center of the spine to nourish and fill the Brain. We can see this process mirrored, to a large degree, when examining the pathways and functions of the *qiao mai*, which start from the Earth and rise up to nourish the head and Brain. Similarly, the Bladder channel is one of the only primary channels that enters the Brain, demonstrating further confluence in the anatomical pathways of the Kidney–Bladder channels and the *qiao mai*.

Lastly, we see correspondences when we look at the ways in which both the Kidney–Bladder system and the *qiao mai* are associated with the nourishment of all of the other *zangfu*, as examined previously. To briefly review this connection, let us look again at what Larre and Rochat de la Vallée write:

> The commentators of the Nan jing and other texts suggest that the *zang* and the innermost are irrigated by the *yin qiao mai*, and the *fu* are watered by the *yang qiao mai*. This is just another way to show the total impregnation in the rising up movement of the *yin* and *yang* of the body. This could be interpreted as the *zang* and the *fu*, or the inner and outer parts of the body, or the front and the back – all interpretations are possible, because the main function of the *qiao mai* is to rule the exchanges and to create equilibrium between the *yin* and the *yang* at every level. (1997, p. 174)

It is clear that the *qiao mai* have a strong relationship to the mobilization of Kidney *yin* and *yang*, in addition to the mobilization of the *jing*-essence and Marrow—just as the Kidney and Bladder primary channels and *zangfu* are directly related to these functional processes. It is also interesting to note the choice of words in the above quotation—that the *yin qiao mai* "irrigates" and the *yang qiao mai* "waters" the *zang* and *fu*, respectively. This languaging clearly draws on underlying associations of the *qiao mai* to the Water element, the Kidneys and Bladder.

If both the *qiao mai* and the Kidney–Bladder system relate to the mobilization of the fundamental *yin* and *yang* within the body—the arising, spreading, and intertwining of *yin* and *yang*—then, in terms of the evolution of consciousness, this is the process of manifestation that occurs once the axis of vertical integration is established. The movement and interplay of *yin* and *yang* occurs once the vertical foundation of the three (Heaven–Humanity–Earth, or *ren–chong–du mai* and Lung–Spleen–Heart) is established, thus allowing the free-flowing interaction of *yin* and *yang* at all levels throughout the individuated being.

The *Wei Mai* and the Pericardium–San Jiao System

After flowing through the Kidney and Bladder channels, the *ying qi* moves into the Pericardium and San Jiao primary channels (corresponding to the time period 7pm–11pm in the horary clock), where it passes the confluent points of the *wei mai*—*neiguan* P-6 and *waiguan* SJ-5. In this section, I examine the correspondences between the *wei mai* and the Pericardium and San Jiao, specifically the ways in which both systems relate to boundaries and the connection between self and other at the level of humanity.

"*Wei*" (維) is often translated as "linking;" thus "*yin wei mai*" is often translated as "Interior Linking Vessel," and *"yang wei mai"* as "Exterior Linking Vessel."[2] As stated by Li Shi Zhen: "Hence, the *yang wei* governs the exterior of the entire body while the *yin wei* governs the interior of the entire body, and so they are referred to as *qian* and *kun*" (Chase and Shima 2010, p. 96). Therefore, the *yin wei mai* functions to link the interior and all of the *yin* meridians, and the *yang wei mai* functions to link the exterior and all of the *yang* meridians; together the *wei mai* are thus able to allow interconnection between the interior and exterior.[3]

Building on this concept, the *wei mai* are often depicted as nets or boundaries. The nature of boundaries is that they simultaneously integrate and separate, determining what is allowed in and what is kept out, and it is through this function that they maintain individual integrity and "hold one together." For this reason, boundaries relate to the pivot between two individuated entities or aspects of being, and have the potential to maintain separateness or transcend the duality to experience oneness. In this case, the *wei mai* form boundaries between the inside and the outside, and self and other. As seen in Chapter 4, the *yin wei mai* relates to the connection and integration within self, an integration of the internal manifestation of the moving polarity of *yin*

---

2   It is interesting to note that the character *"wei"* (維) and the character *"jiao"* (焦) of "San Jiao" are based upon the same character, which has a relation to the idea of linking or attachment—see Larre and Rochat de la Vallée (1997, p. 209) for a fuller discussion on the relationship of these characters.

3   Also see the 27th Difficult Issue, "The yang tie and the yin tie vessels are tied like a network to the body. When they are filled to overflowing, [their contents] stagnate; they cannot [return to the] circulating [influences] by drainage into the [main] conduits. Hence, the yang tie [vessel] originates from a point where all yang [vessels] meet each other, and the yin tie [vessel] originates from a point where all yin [vessels] intersect" (Unschuld 1986, p. 327).

and *yang*; once this integration occurs, one can extend to connect with all else present at the level of humanity. Such extension is a connecting of the exterior, and relates to the function of the *yang wei mai*.

This function of connecting and separating interior and exterior, and self and other, is in perfect resonance with the functions of the Pericardium and San Jiao. The Pericardium in its physical form is often known as the wrapping of the Heart (*xinbao*), which is a wrapping, net, or boundary that simultaneously connects and separates the Heart from everything else around it, thus protecting the Heart from pernicious influences while letting in those things which we hold most dear in our lives and our experiences, those things and people which we "allow into our hearts." Similarly, the San Jiao is often described as the three body cavities, which are boundaries that connect and separate the rest of the internal organs from the periphery and exterior. As written by Hua Tuo in the *Zhong Cang Jing* (Classic of the Secret Transmission), "The Triple Burner...assembles and directs the 5 Yin and 6 Yang organs, the Nutritive and Defensive Qi and the channels, [it harmonizes] the Qi of interior and exterior, left and right, upper and lower" (as cited in Maciocia 2005, p. 88). Clearly, both the Pericardium–San Jiao system and the *wei mai* function as pivots or boundaries between interior and exterior.[4]

---

4   On a side note, it is interesting that *waiguan* SJ-5 is one of the primary points used for any arthritic (*bi*) syndrome. The term arthritis is derived from the Latin "arthros," meaning articulations. Joints are places of articulation, or pivot, between two distinct aspects. This relates to joints at the physical level, but can also be extended to the boundary between Self and Other, which is another form of articulation. Arthritic syndromes are often related to the invasion of external pathogenic

In the five-element tradition, the Pericardium is said to regulate intimate relationships, whereas the San Jiao regulates social relationships. As stated by Jarrett:

> The heart protector is concerned with discerning the appropriate cues for lowering the boundary that limits access both into, and out of, the inner frontier which is the domain of the heart... Compared to the heart protector, the triple heater governs the more social aspects of fire, and gathers and assimilates subtle cues in the environment relevant to the regulation of intimacy. (2004, pp. 217–219)[5]

This offers further support that the Pericardium and San Jiao are boundaries that simultaneously connect and separate individual entities from each other at the horizontal level of manifestation, that they form boundaries in the movement between the inside and outside.

Another interesting correlation arises when examining possible pathways of the *wei mai*. In the contemporary Chinese medical tradition, the pathways of the *wei mai* are vague at best, with no clear consensus about where

---

factors that make their way to the interior; they are then shunted to the joints as a means of preventing it from penetrating to the interior. Thus the joints are a form of pivot, or boundary, between inside and outside.

5   Also see the following citations from Jarrett: "The heart protector and triple heater may be thought of as the guard stations protecting the imperial city and the borders of the country, respectively" (2004, p. 359); "These two points [*neiguan* P-6 and *waiguan* SJ-5] functionally unite the heart protector and three heater officials in a way that empowers the healthy balance of social and intimate relationships" (2004, p. 360).

they start and end (see Appendix).[6] As seen previously, however, it is accepted in certain Daoist traditions that the pathways of the *wei mai* closely parallel the pathways of the Pericardium and San Jiao primary channels. Further, as was seen in the last chapter, the *wei mai* have a relatively stronger correspondence to the arms, while the *qiao mai* have a relatively stronger correspondence to the legs. This demonstrates further resonance between the *qiao mai* with the Kidney and Bladder primary channels (Foot Shaoyin and Foot Taiyang channels, respectively) and the *wei mai* with the Pericardium and San Jiao primary channels (Hand Jueyin and Hand Shaoyang channels, respectively). Further correspondences can be extrapolated when we examine the role of the Pericardium and San Jiao as the Ministerial Fire, when compared with the role of the Heart and Small Intestine as the Emperor Fire—the Ministerial Fire (relating to the Pericardium/San Jiao and *wei mai*, in this model) is responsible for the horizontal axis of integration, connecting with all else that exists at the level of humanity.

---

6   Li Shi Zhen has stated that: "The *yang wei* arises at the meeting of all the yang and travels upward from the outer ankle in the protective aspect; the yin wei arises at the intersection of all the yin and travels upward from the inner ankle in the nutritive aspect, and [together] they constitute a binding network for the entire body" (Chase and Shima 2010, p. 95). As noted by Pirog, "It is not made clear, however, where their exact trajectories lie. The two 'confluences' mentioned in this passage were later interpreted by Li Shi Zhen as UB 63 for the yang wei mai and Ki 9 for the yin wei mai, and these points have been accepted as starting points for the two vessels ever since. Given the location of these two points, they seem unlikely candidates as 'confluences'... Presumably, Li Shi Zhen was following an independent unwritten tradition, as is so often evident in the writings on extraordinary vessels" (1996, p. 202).

We can also examine the pathologies associated with the *wei mai* and the Pericardium–San Jiao system. One of the primary pathologies of the *yin wei mai* is heartache. Heart pain is also one of the primary signs of a Pericardium issue; thus it makes sense that *neiguan* P-6 is one of the pre-eminent points for any form of Heart pain.[7] Not only is it the confluent point of the *yin wei mai* and a point along the Pericardium channel, it is also the *luo*-connecting point—and it therefore assists in the re-integration of *yin* and *yang* and may help to re-establish appropriate boundaries within self.

Similarly, the pathology associated with the *yang wei mai* has resonance to the San Jiao. According to the *Nan Jing* (Classic of Difficult Issues): "When the yang tie has an illness, one suffers from [fits of] cold and heat" (Unschuld 1986, p. 333). Chills and fever are seen primarily in exterior pathologies, when the *wei qi* and the outermost level of the body is being affected—thus offering confirmation of the *yang wei mai* as one of the outermost boundaries, much as the San Jiao is one of the outermost boundaries of the *zangfu* organs. Similarly, alternating chills and fever are one of the primary indications of a *shaoyang* stage imbalance; the San Jiao is the channel of hand *shaoyang*, and points along the San Jiao primary channel are often used for such disorders.

---

7   Also see Larre and Rochat de la Vallée: "The heart is the deepest and most important dwelling place for the unity. It is the residence of the spirits and the place which attracts the special concentration of essences coming from all the other *zang*. The heart is also the master of the psychological world, the emotions and sentiments, so it is also master of the upper orifices and sense organs because, acting as a master, it has to make decisions based on the information coming from outside. We can use this unity in order to have a curative effect for our patients" (2003, p. 64).

The *Dai Mai* and the Liver and Gall Bladder System

Returning to the horary clock, the *ying qi* finishes up its daily cycle with the Gall Bladder and Liver primary channels. This corresponds to the time period 11pm–3am, during which time the *ying qi* passes *zulinqi* GB-41, confluent point of the *dai mai*. Many of the connections and correspondences between the *dai mai* and the Liver–Gall Bladder system have been covered in previous chapters, so here I will only briefly summarize some of the major points relevant to this discussion.

Zulinqi GB-41 is the confluent point of the *dai mai* as well as the exit point of the Gall Bladder channel, as noted above. Thus it is the place where the *ying qi* leaves the Gall Bladder channel to connect with the Liver channel during the horary cycle, suggesting that the *dai mai* may share in this connection between the Gall Bladder and Liver channels—similar in many ways to the actions of *luo*-connecting points. Further, in the proposed theoretical framework pairing the extraordinary vessels with the extraordinary *fu*, the *dai mai* and Gall Bladder are paired together, as they have strong correspondences to each other—functionally, anatomically, and evolutionarily.

Another significant correspondence between the *dai mai* and Liver–Gall Bladder system is in the relationship they both have to transition/transcendence, the movement from the end of one cycle to the start of the next. In the daily evolutionary cycle of the extraordinary vessels, we explored the ways in which the *dai mai* may function to take one from the most exteriorized/manifest state all the way back to the deepest quiescence, to the lower *dantian* and the *ren–chong–du mai*. Similarly, the Gall Bladder, which pertains to the *zangfu* organ system as well as doubling as an extraordinary *fu*, provides a means to connect post-heaven back to pre-heaven. We also see this theme continued when examining the place of the Gall Bladder and Liver primary channels along the horary clock—they are the last primary channels of the horary clock through which the *ying qi* cycles on a daily basis, before returning to the Lung channel to start the cycle over again the next day. They therefore function to bring us back to the beginning, and to continue the cycle anew each day.

The Horizontal Axis, Manifestation, and Transcendence

Just as the first six primary channels of the horary clock and the extraordinary vessels that form the quiescent state share an intimate relationship to the vertical axis, so too it is clear that the second six primary channels and their paired extraordinary vessels share an intimate relationship to the horizontal axis, manifestation, and transcendence. We can see the processes of the horizontal axis and manifestation/connection demonstrated in the functions and correspondences of the *qiao mai* and Kidney–Bladder (manifestation) and the *wei mai* and Pericardium–San Jiao (connection between interior and exterior, self and other). As noted above, both the *qiao mai* and the Kidney–Bladder system relate to the dynamic polarity of *yin* and *yang* as it manifests throughout the body, nourishing the *zangfu* and creating the connection between Earth and the lower *dantian* and Heaven and the upper *dantian*. Thus they have a direct relationship to the process of manifestation in the evolution of consciousness, the coming together and interweaving of Heaven and Earth, body and spirit, *jing* and *shen*.

Similarly, we saw above how the *wei mai* and the Pericardium–San Jiao system have a direct relationship to the connection between interior and exterior, and self and other. Thus the *qiao mai* and *wei mai*, as well as the Kidneys–Bladder and Pericardium–San Jiao, have intimate relationships to the horizontal axis and manifestation. Finally, the *dai mai* and Liver–Gall Bladder system are a direct reflection of the process of transcendence, of connecting post-heaven and duality back to pre-heaven and the quiescent state of oneness.

Through these processes, we see a clear correlation between the primary channels/*zangfu* and the extraordinary vessels with the evolution of consciousness. The first half of the horary clock corresponds to the establishment of the vertical axis of integration within the body, the triad of Heaven, Earth, and Humanity. Once this triad is established, we have the process of manifestation reflected in the Kidney–Bladder system and the *qiao mai*. Once the dynamic polarity of *yin* and *yang* is created, one is able to integrate these dynamic aspects within self, at the level of the Heart and the middle *dantian*, as represented by the *yin wei mai* and the Pericardium. After the internal integration, one is able to connect with all else present at the level of humanity, as represented by the *yang wei mai* and the San Jiao. The final stage in the evolution of consciousness is transcendence of duality and the return to oneness, as represented by the *dai mai* and the Gall Bladder–Liver system.

Conclusion

As explored in this chapter, there is strong evidence to suggest a direct connection between the *zangfu* organ and primary channel systems with the extraordinary vessels. Not only are the confluent points of the extraordinary vessels perfectly distributed among the primary channels, but there are also a number of clear anatomical, functional, and relational correspondences between each system of *zangfu* organ and primary channel pairs and their associated extraordinary vessels. Beyond these correspondences, each system reflects the vertical and horizontal axes and the processes of Daoist cosmogenesis and the evolution of consciousness

The *zangfu* and primary channel pairs are *yin–yang* complements of a whole; they exist at the level of duality and relate to manifestation and day-to-day living. However, all that exists at the level of duality is rooted in the primal unity; thus there is something that precedes them, and that transcends their duality to reconnect to the original unity. It seems clear that the extraordinary vessels underlie and transcend the duality of the *zangfu* organ and primary channel pairs, and are the direct connection that links the manifest duality with the original unity.

CONCLUSION

"Wherever the art of Medicine is loved,
there is also a love of Humanity."

Hippocrates

Life is extraordinary. The very fact that we exist as complex, multidimensional beings at this manifest level, and get to experience—through our senses—others, the world around us, as well as our own selves, is a miracle. Ironically, it is only by existing as individuated beings that we can experience life in this way, and yet it is precisely this individuation that also gives rise to all experience of suffering and feelings of disconnection. All too often it is easy to forget how extraordinary we are, how extraordinary each one of our patients is, and how we are all inherently connected to an underlying and transcendent unity even as we exist as individuated beings at the level of duality. What I have intended in this book is not simply to postulate a nifty theoretical model; if the model is useful for demonstrating correlations and deepening the theoretical understanding of this beautiful medicine, that is wonderful—but the main point I have hoped to highlight is the way in which the model demonstrates a continual unity underlying our experience at the level of humanity.

Once we are incarnated in a body, there is a constant, daily connection to, and movement to return to, the oneness of Heaven, to the *dao*. Through the model presented in this book, it becomes clear that, on a diurnal basis, the order in which the *ying qi* flows through the primary channels accesses the extraordinary vessels and extraordinary organs in such a way as to continually reconnect us to the underlying unity. This is reflected in the movement from Earth to Humanity to Heaven, from lower, to middle, to upper *dantian*, and from legs, to arms, to head. This not only allows each of us to continually maintain our connection to Heaven; additionally, when one is connected in this way, the body has a nearly unlimited capacity to heal itself. When the *qi* flows freely through the body, excesses will naturally be carried off and deficiencies filled, and the body's innate drive towards harmony and connection is maintained.

What is it that is so "extraordinary" about the extraordinary vessels? They relate to the deep, constitutional aspects of self, to the ability for adaptation, growth, development, and transformation. They are reservoirs that can be drawn upon in times of difficulty and crisis, and through this have a direct relationship to the evolution of consciousness. Although it is a natural part of being human to want to avoid suffering, sometimes suffering is unavoidable; often it is precisely during the challenging and extraordinary times of suffering and crisis that we are offered some of the greatest opportunities for growth and development.

During these times, the extraordinary vessels can help ground us in the Source, to remind us of who we are and what we are here for, and to help transition from one developmental stage or way of being to another. In so doing, not only can they allow us to move through challenge, difficulty, and suffering with a greater degree of grace and ease, but they can also help us to gain as much compassion, wisdom, and humanity from such experiences as possible. They accomplish all of this through maintaining our connection to the underlying Source—the oneness that transcends the manifest duality where all suffering occurs. Thus, the extraordinary vessels may be seen as a connection between the microcosm of the human body and the macrocosm of the universe, keeping each individual immersed in the larger system so that irregularities and disequilibrium may be balanced out, and growth can continually occur.

The extraordinary vessels not only help in times of transformation and crisis because they are able to connect us to the Source and the essence, but through this connection are able to give us perspective and help us to feel safe and contained when going through these "extraordinary times" of transformation and crisis. This is often one of the most important aspects of healing—remembering who we are, what we are here for, and what we are doing. Fundamentally, the primary purpose of being human is to connect Heaven and Earth and the inside and the outside; through residing at the pivot of these polarities, the individual can have an experience of unity and oneness, of connection to the *dao*, while existing as a limited, individuated being at the level of duality, and thus experientially exist in the natural state. The extraordinary vessels and organs are one means to have this experience, whether they are accessed through acupuncture, *qigong*, or meditation utilizing these vessels.

The diurnal cycle of the *ying qi* through the primary channels is the key to unlocking the connection between the extraordinary vessels, the extraordinary *fu*, and Daoist conceptions of the evolution of consciousness. The *ying qi* is the middle, or pivot, between the *wei qi* and *jing qi*, and therefore it corresponds to the level of humanity and is at the pivot of various *yin–yang* aspects of being. If the *ying qi* flows freely through the channels, the theoretical model presented here indicates not only that *yin* and *yang* will be in harmony, but that the flow of *ying qi* through the primary channel system will naturally activate the extraordinary vessels and *fu*—allowing them to unfold in the order which reflects the evolution of consciousness— thereby connecting the individual back to the Source and transcending the mundane duality.

The Art of Being Human

In becoming an individuated being at the level of humanity, one is "taking on the burden of being human." What is the burden of being human? It is the burden of connecting Heaven and Earth and expressing love at the level of humanity. For this reason, a closely related Chinese word of the character *ren* (任) (as in the *ren mai*, which etymologically connotes taking on the burden of being human) is *ren* (仁), which is composed of the radical for person with the number "2." While this character is often translated as benevolence, etymologically it is related to expressing care from one person to another, or between two people. Confucius stated that it could be defined as *ai* (愛)—love. Another etymological interpretation of it is that it is the result of an individual person connecting Heaven and Earth.

This suggests that the highest expression of being human is to express love—as embodied wisdom and compassion—at the level of humanity. In so doing, one becomes an emperor—one who connects Heaven and Earth with all of humanity. This is the art of being human—to connect above and below and the inside and the outside, and to experience and express one's humanity is, ultimately, the motive force underlying love, compassion, and wisdom. Love is the highest external manifestation of internal being, and the route that becomes the deepest way in which the external can be experienced internally. This is our natural state as human beings, something that we all have access to, at all times. When one is not in this state, or when one is further from this state, it indicates the presence of blockages within the meridian system that are preventing the full interpenetration of *yin* and *yang* at the level of humanity.

Thus, the primary work we have as humans is to connect Heaven and Earth, and the natural outcome of such a connection is to express love or benevolence between self and other. This is, ultimately, the primary work—the primary "burden"—that we have as incarnated beings at the level of humanity, as well as the means to cultivate and express our humanity. As stated by Han Yu (768–824), "Universal love is called humanity. To practice this in the proper manner is called righteousness. To proceed according to these is called the Tao" (as cited in

Chan 1963, p. 454). It is not that we need to cultivate humanity because it is "good" or because we "should"; being in touch with suffering—our own as well as that of others—is the only way to become whole within ourselves, to become more fully human and accomplish what we are here for. Cultivating humanity entails cultivating humility, presence, and compassion; in care giving, we come face to face with suffering, with the pain of others, and are thus given an incredible opportunity to cultivate humanity—our own as well as that of our patients.

Humanity occurs at the level of the heart; the heart is the human-level reality, centered between Heaven and Earth. To be fully human is to be conscious of and to realize one's connectedness to everything and everyone else, and to make decisions and take action based on the reality of each moment and not on pre-conditioned values or realities. As stated by David Frawley and Vasant Lad, "True humanity, which is humane feeling for all life, is at the heart of all life... It is only when we come to look upon all things as human that we are capable of a truly humane existence" (1986, p. 3).

Residing at the pivot of any *yin–yang* polarity gives rise to the moment of experiential awareness. Therefore, to be "centered within oneself" is to be residing at the pivot between upper and lower, inside and outside, body and spirit, *yin* and *yang*. All of the pivots within the body relate—energetically, functionally, and spatially—to the ability to be fully, experientially present in the moment. For it is at the pivot of any given duality that one has the opportunity to transcend duality—which includes the dualities of vertical and horizontal, self and other, and space and time. The *chong mai* is the pivot between *ren* and *du mai*, as well as pre-heaven and post-heaven; the middle *dantian* is the pivot between the upper and lower *dantian*; the individuated human is a pivot between Heaven and Earth and the inside and the outside.

Pre-heaven *qi* comes from the stored essence and provides the basis for experiencing at the level of humanity; post-heaven *qi* comes from digesting that which we consume/experience. Heaven lies between these two; therefore, Heaven is the moment of experiential awareness. The act of consciously experiencing allows one to reside at the pivot, which allows one to reside in Heaven—that is, a state of unity. In digesting one's experiences, one generates post-heaven *qi*. The more an individual allows themselves to fully experience each moment, the greater the efficiency with which each experience will produce post-heaven *qi*, and the more energy/vitality will grow. The greater the production of post-heaven *qi*, the easier it becomes to replenish and store up pre-heaven *qi*. After experiencing and producing post-heaven *qi*, the reverse alchemical process occurs as this is brought down, condensed, and converted to essence—which then becomes pre-heaven *qi* for future experiential moments. For this reason, it can be suggested that the act of consciously experiencing produces *qi* and essence, and occurs when one is in—as well as causes one to be in—the natural state.

The natural state is our birthright, as well as what we are here for. It is through moving closer to the natural state that we actualize our destiny. However, simply because we all have the natural state within us does not mean that we actualize it all the time. We all have struggles, trauma, and blockages simply from being human and living a human life on earth, and these challenges will often pull us out of our experiential awareness of the natural state. The key, however, is to recognize that all of these are simply obscurations that cover over the brilliance of our true beauty; the natural state is always there within, waiting for us to recognize it.

The practice of medicine is always based on an underlying cosmology, a perspective on humanity, who we are, and what we are here for. The model put forth in this book demonstrates that, from the perspective of Daoism and Chinese medicine, every human being is inextricably linked to Heaven above and Earth below, and that we have access to this connection every single day at all times, through the extraordinary vessels and organs. Shifting our perspective has the ability to change how we practice the medicine. If we change our assumptions about reality, and the meaning of suffering, it will actually change how we interact with our patients, and it will change how we apply the therapeutic methods that we have at our disposal.

There is a continuum between medicine, healing, and spirituality; part of the role of any practitioner of medicine is to understand how to manage the spectrum between healing and self-actualization, between remedying physical maladies and encouraging spiritual growth. For this reason, the art of practicing medicine is not merely to "fix" problems or discomforts, but to help our patients to become more whole in all senses, and thus to help them move closer to the natural state.

Appendix

PATHWAYS OF THE
EXTRAORDINARY VESSELS

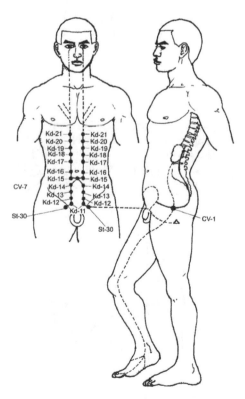

The Chong channel

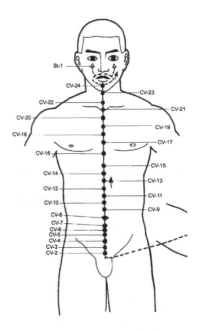

The Ren channel

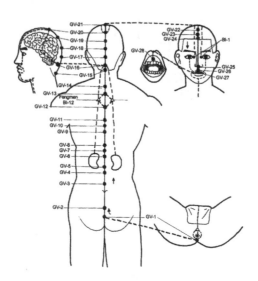

The Du channel

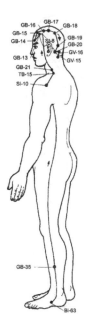

The Yang Wei channel

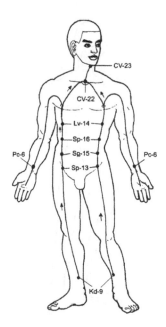

The Yin Wei channel

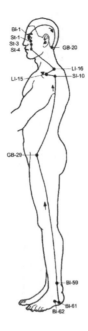

The Yang Qiao channel

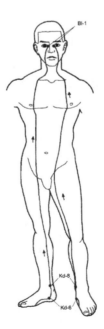

The Yin Qiao channel

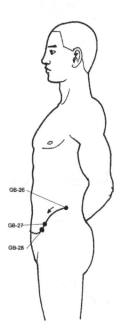

The Dai Mai channel

REFERENCES

Allan, Sarah. (1997). *The Way of Water and Sprouts of Virtue*. Albany: State University of New York Press.

Chan, Wing-Tsit, ed. (1963). *A Source Book in Chinese Philosophy*. Princeton: Princeton University Press.

Chase, Charles and Miki Shima. (2010). *An Exposition on the Eight Extraordinary Vessels: Acupuncture, Alchemy, and Herbal Medicine*. Seattle: Eastland Press.

Deadman, Peter and Mazin Al-Khafaji, with Kevin Baker. (2005). *A Manual of Acupuncture* (revised ed.). East Sussex: Journal of Chinese Medicine Publications.

Deng, Ming-Dao. (1990). *Scholar Warrior: An Introduction to the Tao in Everyday Life*. New York: HarperCollins.

The Encyclopedia of Taoism. (2008). Fabrizio Pregadio, ed. New York: Routledge.

Frawley, David and Vasant Lad. (1986). *The Yoga of Herbs: An Ayurvedic Guide to Herbal Medicine*. Twin Lakes: Lotus Press.

Harbaugh, Rick. (1999). *Chinese Characters: A Genealogy and Dictionary*. New Haven: Yale University Press.

Harper, Donald. (2001). "Iatromancy, Diagnosis, and Prognosis in Early Chinese Medicine." In Elisabeth Hsu, ed., *Innovation in Chinese Medicine*. Cambridge: Cambridge University Press.

Jarrett, Lonny. (2004). *Nourishing Destiny: The Inner Tradition of Chinese Medicine*. Stockbridge: Spirit Path Press.

Kohn, Livia. (1989a). "Guarding the One: Concentrative Meditation in Taoism." In Livia Kohn, ed., *Taoist Meditation and Longevitiy Techniques*. Ann Arbor: University of Michigan Press.

Kohn, Livia. (1989b) "Taoist Insight Meditation: The Tang Practice of "Neiguan."" In Liva Kohn, ed., *Taoist Meditation and Longevitiy Techniques*. Ann Arbor: University of Michigan Press.

Larre, Claude and Elisabeth Rochat de la Vallée. (1997). *The Eight Extraordinary Meridians*. Cambridge: Monkey Press. Transcribed and edited by Sandra Hill.

Larre, Claude and Elisabeth Rochat de la Vallée. (2003). *The Extraordinary Fu*. Cambridge: Monkey Press.

Lee, Miriam. (1992). *Insights of a Senior Acupuncturist*. Boulder: Blue Poppy Press.

Lo, Vivienne. (2001). "The Influence of Nurturing Life Culture on the Development of Western Han Acumoxa Therapy." In Elisabeth Hsu, ed., *Innovation in Chinese Medicine*. Cambridge: Cambridge University Press.

Maciocia, Giovanni. (2005). *Foundations of Chinese Medicine: A Comprehensive Text for Acupuncturists and Herbalists* (2nd ed.). London: Churchill Livingstone.

Matsumoto, Kiiko and Stephen Birch. (1986). *Extraordinary Vessels*. Brookline: Paradigm Publications.

Mi, Huang-Fu. (2004). *Jia Yi Jing* (The Systematic Classic of Acupuncture and Moxibustion). Translated by Yang Shou-Zhong and Charles Chace. Boulder: Blue Poppy Press.

Morris, William. (2002a). "Pulse Diagnosis Using the Elemental Compass Model." *Acupuncture Today*, 3, 8.

Morris, William. (2002b). "Eight Extra Vessel Pulse Diagnosis: A Path to Effective Treatment." *Acupuncture Today*, 3, 1.

Morris, William. (2009). *Chinese Pulse Diagnosis: Epistemology, Practice, and Tradition* (Doctoral Dissertation). Available from Dissertations and Theses database. (UMI No. 3350675).

Mu, Wang. (2011). *The Foundations of Internal Alchemy: The Taoist Practice of Neidan*. Translated by Fabrizio Pregadio. Mountain View: Golden Elixir Press.

Needham, Joseph with Lu Gwei-djin. (1966). "Medicine and Chinese Culture." In Mansel Davies, ed. (1990) *A Selection from the Writings of Joseph Needham*. Sussex: The Book Guild.

Ni, Maoshing. (1995). *The Yellow Emperor's Classic of Medicine: A New Translation of the Neijing Suwen with Commentary.* Boston: Shambhala.

Pirog, John. (1996). *The Practical Application of Meridian Style Acupuncture.* Berkeley: Pacific View Press.

Pregadio, Fabrizio. (2015). "An Introduction to Daoism." Accessed on 2/12/18 at: www.goldenelixir.com/taoism/taoism_intro_5.html.

Richardson, Thomas. (2008). "The Natural State." *The Empty Vessel: A Journal of Contemporary Taoism,* 15, 2.

Richardson, Thomas. (2009a). "The Dai Mai: Dynamic Structural Stability and Spherical Integration." *The American Acupuncturist,* 48.

Richardson, Thomas. (2009b). "The Ying Qi Cycle and the Diurnal Evolutionary Unfoldment of the Extraordinary Vessels." *California Journal of Oriental Medicine,* 20, 2.

Richardson, Thomas. (2010a). "Vertical and Horizontal Integration: The Dynamic Flow of *Qi* at the Level of Humanity." *The Lantern,* 7, 2.

Richardson, Thomas. (2010b). "Pairing the Extraordinary Vessels and the Extraordinary Fu – Part 2: The Ying Qi Cycle and The Evolution of Consciousness." *Chinese Medicine Times,* 5, 2.

Richardson, Thomas. (2010c). "Pairing the Extraordinary Vessels and the Extraordinary *Fu.*" *Chinese Medicine Times,* 5, 1.

Richardson, Thomas. (2011). "Pairing the Extraordinary Vessels with the Primary Channels and *Zangfu,* Part 1." *Chinese Medicine Times,* 6, 3.

Richardson, Thomas. (2012a). "The *Ying Qi* Cycle and a Relation of the Extraordinary Vessels to Daoist Cosmology." *The Lantern: A Journal of Traditional Chinese Medicine,* 9, 1.

Richardson, Thomas. (2012b). "Pairing the Extraordinary Vessels with the Primary Channels and Zangfu, Part 2." *Chinese Medicine Times,* 7, 1.

Richardson, Thomas. (2014). "The Natural State: Daoist and Chinese Medical Views." *The Lantern: A Journal of Traditional Chinese Medicine,* 11, 3.

Richardson, Thomas. (2015)."Medicine as Metaphor." *Acupuncture Today,* 16, 8.

Roth, Harold D. (1999). *Original Tao: Inward Training (Nei-Yeh) and the Foundations of Taoist Mysticism.* New York: Columbia University Press.

Salguero, Pierce. (2013). "'On Eliminating Disease': Translations of the Medical Chapter from the Chinese Versions of the Sutra of the Golden Light." *eJournal of Indian Medicine* 6, 1: 21–43.

Unschuld, Paul. (1986). *Nan-Ching: The Classic of Difficult Issues*. Berkeley: University of California Press.

Wang, Bing. (1997). *Yellow Emperor's Canon of Internal Medicine*. Translated by N.L. Wu and A.Q. Wu. Beijing: China Science & Technology Press.

Wong, Eva (Translator). (1992). *Cultivating Stillness: A Taoist Manual for Transforming Body and Mind*. Boston: Shambhala Publications.

Wong, K. Chimin and Lien-Teh Wu. (1932). *History of Chinese Medicine*. Tientsin, China: The Tientsin Press.

Wu, Jing-Nuan. (1993). *Ling Shu* (The Spiritual Pivot). Honolulu: University of Hawai'i Press.

Yang, Rur-Bin. (2003). "From 'Merging the Body with the Mind' to 'Wandering in Unitary Qi 氣': A Discussion of *Zhuangzi's* Realm of the True Man and Its Corporeal Basis." *Hiding the World in the World: Uneven Discourses on the Zhuangzi*, ed. Scott Cook. Albany: State University of New York Press.

Yuen, Jeffrey. (2005). *Channel Systems of Chinese Medicine: The Eight Extraordinary Vessels*. Transcript from seminar held 12–13 April 2003, New England School of Acupuncture, Continuing Education Department. Edited by Stephen Howard.

Yuen, Jeffrey. (2006). *The Curious Organs (Qi Heng Zhi Fu): Including Energetics and Pathology, Treatment Protocols, and Selected Characters*. Transcripts from seminar held 21–22 June 2003, New England School of Acupuncture, Continuing Education Department. Edited by Stephen Howard.

INDEX